STRONG
AT EVERYTHING
WEAK at
NOTHING

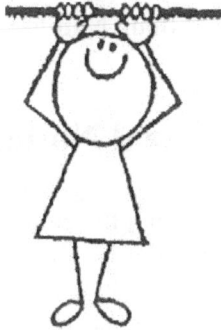

How to __MOTIVATE YOUR KIDS__ to:

- **Eat Better**
- **Exercise More**
- **Immunize Themselves Against Obesity for Life!**

By
Rick and Pam Osbourne

Copyright Notices

Legal Notices

"When you dream a dream alone, it's only a dream.

When you dream a dream together, it's reality!"

...John Lennon

How To Win Their Hearts…

"Do you know how to win a five year old boy's heart? Well, you drop down to one knee, look him right in the eye, and listen as if what he's telling you is really important…cause it is.

And if you happen to speak at all, whatever you say from that position will be infinitely better than anything you can possibly say from on high.

Oh, and by the way, five year old girls? They're just the same."

> …A wise old teacher/coach somewhere,
> sometime, someplace

"I try never to look down on those who look up to me."

…Muhammad Ali

This book is dedicated to
all those kids who want to be

Strong at Everything and
Weak at Nothing!

Table of Contents

                                                            Page

The American Society of Exercise Physiologists   7

The 12 Core Concepts of OPYOW   9

The Foundations of OPYOW   13
1. OPYOW as a Philosophy of Education   14
2. An Old Coach Offers a Simple Solution   16
3. Strong at Everything, Weak at Nothing   20
4. OPYOW: 5 Goals and 7 Habits   23
5. OPYOW: 7 Basic Presumptions   25
6. OPYOW: Enlightened Self Interest   27
7. What do You Expect Kids to Learn?   30
8. Privilege VS Obligation   32
9. The Missing Ingredient   34
10. Many Virtues of Infinite Measurability   38
11. Mother Nature Defines Fitness   41

The Mechanics of OPYOW   47
1. A Nuts and Bolts Explanation With Photos   48
2. Functional Body Composition Testing   54
3. Functional Fitness: Functional Beauty   57
4. Functional Performance Testing   59
5. Coach, I Can't Do Pull-ups. What Now?   61
6. Conventional VS Leg Assisted Pull-ups   63
7. OPYOW With a Jump Rope   65

The Motivational Psychology of OPYOW   69
1. Motivating Kids to Take Action Today   70
2. The Most Important Lesson Kids Can Learn   73
3. What Happens When the Going Gets Tough?   78
4. Embarrassed When Talking About Obesity?   81
5. No You Can't: Yes I Can   84
6. Motivating Through Public Success   86
7. Using What Kids Want to Motivate Them   88

8. Selling Cool: Winning the War on Obesity   91
9. Some Want to be Bad: None Want to be Weak   93
10. An Open Letter to Kids   95
11. Instant and Delayed Gratification   98
12. ROI and Compound Interest of Fitness   100
13. Rufus, the Natural Born Runner   102
14. My Motivation   105

OPYOW: The Appendix   **107**
1. The OPYOW Strong/Weak Test   108
2. The Strong/Weak Food Test   111
3. Strong Table VS Weak Table   114
4. Great Publicity   115
5. The Democratic Effects of OPYOW   117
6. A Cost Effective Plan for Schools   119
7. A Salute to Relentless Persistence   122
8. An Open Letter to President Obama   125
9. Obama and the OPYOW Challenge   128
10. Obesity and the Future of Democracy   130
11. One is Never a Statistic   132
12. Boiling it Down: a Common Denominator   134
13. A Form Letter for People of Action   137
14. The Logistics of OPYOW   140
15. Organizing OPYOW in PE Class   144
16. How Important is Confidence?   148
17. The World is Shaped by People of Action   150
18. The OPYOW Pledge   152
19. OPYOW: A Disclaimer   153

The American Society of Exercise Physiologists Endorses FATS as a Simple Solution to Childhood Obesity

Duluth, MN – Performance in exercises in which the participant's own body weight is the primary resistance (i.e. pull-ups, push ups, dips, and hand stand push ups) automatically improves when the participant loses enough body fat because the workload is reduced. For example, a 150 lb. person who loses 25 lbs. would find it much easier to do pull-ups, jump higher, or run faster because they're carrying 16% less resistance. By the same token, the performance of a 150 lb. person who gains 25 lbs. of body fat will deteriorate because the workload has increased.

Exercises that use extrinsic, non-body weight resistance, (i.e. weights, plates, springs, and rubber bands) don't enjoy the same automatic performance feedback. Your bench press, for example, won't automatically change just because you lost or gained 25 lbs. of fat.

Functional Acid Test Strategy (FATS)

This simple recognition has led to a new acronym in the field of childhood obesity prevention. Ironically it's called FATS which stands for *Functional Acid Test Strategy*. In the words of American Society of Exercise Physiologists President and former collegiate gymnast Dr. Tommy Boone, "Certain body weight exercises are challenging enough that obese people can't do them. Pull-ups, dips, and handstand push ups, for example, fall into that category."

One Example of FATS

So the FATS strategy suggests that a child choose one of those challenging body weight exercises as their own *functional acid test*, and then learn to master it. One example is a program called **Operation Pull Your Own Weight** which says, "Kids who can do pull-ups are never obese. If you start them early, before they've had a chance to gain much weight, most kids can learn to do pull-ups in a predictable amount of time. And once they've learned to do pull-ups, they're immunized against obesity for life, as long as they maintain the ability." A simpler, more cost effective solution to childhood obesity would be hard to imagine.

Focusing on the Positive

The beauty of the FATS orientation is that it focuses on a child's strength development (all kids want to be strong at everything) instead of focusing on the negative and embarrassing concept of fat loss. With this extremely positive approach kids see it as cool, they buy in, and in a predictable period of time they can *naturally immunize themselves against obesity for life*.

Simple, Easily Documented, and Affordable

In Boone's words, "At ASEP we endorse active lifestyles and nutritious eating habits across the board. But we believe that the simplicity and positive character of the FATS orientation to childhood obesity prevention has something special to bring to this long and frustrating debate. It could be what we've been looking for all along. It's simple, easily implemented, documented, and affordable. Those kinds of assets are hard to beat these days."

OPYOW: The 12 Core Concepts

1. **Motivation:** According to its practitioners, the three most important factors in real estate are location, location, and location. According to its practitioners, the three most important things in fitness (and probably in life) are motivation, motivation, and motivation. With that said, EVERYTHING in this book is related to the subject of motivation. It's completely and totally about MOTIVATION!!!

2. **Strong at Everything, Weak at Nothing:** This little phrase represents the philosophical foundation of this book because we contend that all kids, from 3 to 93, want to be strong at everything. We've also never met even one kid who wants to be weak at anything. So this book is also all about getting strong…in all kinds of ways.

3. **Opportunity vs. Obligation:** We've observed that there's a huge difference between *those things we get to do, and those things we have to do*. In fact the things we *get to do*, or *actively choose to do* are always more valuable to us than anything *we have to do*. For that reason we never force any kid to participate in OPYOW because that reduces its value dramatically. Treating OPYOW as an *opportunity* instead of an *obligation* is an essential ingredient to the mix.

4. **Winning and Self Competition:** Winning in OPYOW happens WHENEVER <u>YOU</u> IMPROVE. In other words, whenever you become even a little stronger, that's a reason to celebrate winning. And if you do it every day, winning becomes a habit regardless of what anyone else is doing.

5. **Small, Regular Increments of Progress:** The journey of a thousand miles starts with a single step. It's a huge mistake to expect to make progress in large chunks. It's a motivation killer. That's why the opportunity for kids to make small but

regular increments of progress over time is absolutely essential in OPYOW.

6. **Public Success**: There are two great motivators in OPYOW. The first is regular, tangible progress which constitutes personal winning. The second is the recognition and celebration of these successes by one's peers. When one rubs up against the other on a regular basis over time, motivation blooms and becomes imbedded in the participant's DNA forever. That constitutes a huge win!

7. **Relentless Persistence**: When a child is motivated to become strong, is given the opportunity to do so, experiences progress on a regular basis in public in front of their peers, and motivation becomes imbedded in their DNA, the inevitable result is that they become relentlessly persistent in this natural habit of growth. When relentless persistence takes root, you're operating on a different level and winning becomes more than probable, it becomes inevitable.

8. **Function vs. Cosmetics**: OPYOW is all about what you can do as opposed to what you look like. Winning is something that must be earned as opposed to something you can purchase at the cosmetic counter. Beauty itself is defined and understood in functional terms like athleticism and physical grace, and is a quality that can be achieved by most people regardless of their genetic inheritance.

9. **Five Goals:** In OPYOW we have five goals including: compete with yourself, to be a little stronger this week than last week, to be a little stronger this month than last month, and to be a lot stronger this year than last year, and to be able to do at least one legitimate pull-up, and ideally a lot more.

10. **Seven Habits:** In OPYOW we recognize seven habits that make you stronger on the pull-up bar and in every other way. They include: regular work, eating right, getting sufficient rest, avoiding tobacco, avoiding alcohol, avoiding drugs, and

taking responsibility for yourself because nobody else can do that for you.

11. **Enlightened Self Interest** – OPYOW presumes that you have to be strong enough yourself before you can help anyone else become strong. But where individual strength has limits, the opportunity to help others get strong is unlimited, and in this sense one's own strength can be multiplied exponentially over and over again. Becoming strong yourself is level one. Helping others become strong is level two and represents the black belt of OPYOW.

12. **Accessibility/Practicality** – One of the most significant core concepts of OPYOW is that anything that's going to succeed with childhood obesity has to be simple, documentable, easily accessible, and ultimately practical. In this sense simplicity is OPYOW's greatest strength. It also requires almost no space, almost no budget, almost no time (30 kids can workout twice, in about an hour per week). And documentation is a piece of cake

And in the End...

In this book you'll find these twelve core concepts woven in and around each other in various ways, in various contexts and combinations, and approached from various angles. If you have a practical grip on them, however, you will know how, and you will be able to successfully motivate your kids to eat better, exercise more, and to naturally immunize themselves against obesity for life.

And if you're motivated enough and you're relentlessly persistent enough to read this book from cover to cover, by the time you're finished you will have a practical grip on these twelve core concepts. And when you do, you'll have a uniquely practical knowledge to offer your own kids, and your community, and anyone else who's privileged enough to work with you.

The Remainder of the Book

It's worth recognizing that since each one of these chapters have been written to be independent, stand-on-their-own articles, they can be read in almost any order and still make sense.

However in the name of organization, the remainder of the book has been divided into four specific sections, including OPYOW's Foundations, Mechanics, Psychological Motivation, and Appendix. Anything that was important enough to include, but failed to fit neatly into one of the first three sections was placed in the Appendix. Now feel please free to dig in.

The Foundations of

Operation Pull Your Own Weight

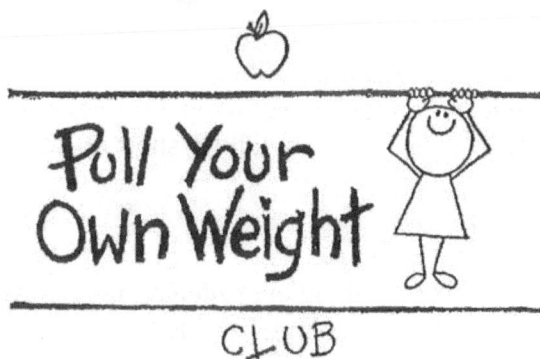

Pull Your
Own Weight

CLUB

Pull Your Own Weight as a Philosophy of Education

Strong VS Weak

We believe it's the nature of all kids to want to be strong at everything and weak at nothing. In other words, you'll meet plenty of kids these days who are proud of "being bad." But you won't meet any who are proud of "being weak" at anything.

We believe that given the right conditions, almost all kids NATURALLY become a little stronger mentally, spiritually, and physically, every day, every week, every month, and every year. And if those strength gains are documented and celebrated publicly, in front of family and friends, these kids will soon *learn to expect success* instead of failure.

Returns on Their Investments

They'll also learn that there's a payoff, a return on their investment of time and effort, and that with relentless persistence they can tackle difficult tasks one bite at a time, and expect to succeed in almost anything. You see, most kids never learn this lesson and so most kids inevitably fall far short of fulfilling their true potential.

Opportunity VS Obligation

We believe that anything presented as an opportunity (you *get* to do it) will become more highly valued than anything presented as an obligation (you *have* to do it). And in this opportunistic light, real education (growing stronger) becomes highly valued and it ignites a kid's desire to participate. On the other hand when something is mandated and kids are obligated to participate, it undermines any genuine motivation, and failure wins by default. It becomes the proverbial self fulfilling prophecy.

Systematically Undermining Motivation and Self Confidence

Finally we believe that kids come to school at various levels of maturity and development, and requiring them to compete against each other at a young age is a sure fire way to de-motivate the highest percentage of them who, for all kinds of silly reasons, are variously labeled average, below average, or much worse, by a system that's inadvertently designed to undermine the kids it actually wants to support.

Along with bursting their young motivational bubbles, the system simultaneously strips kids of the self confidence necessary to tackle new challenges and to grow stronger in all kinds of ways. In other words, when motivation and self confidence are systematically (even if inadvertently) undermined, students stop trying. And when they stop trying, failure automatically steps in and becomes the self fulfilling prophecy mentioned above.

The Price of Being Cool

Then again, when their failure is inevitably paraded in front of family and friends, these kids are prepared with the ready made excuse, "I didn't try." You see when you try hard in public, you risk being humiliated…the opposite of being cool. That's a price that a great many kids are unwilling to pay.

The Natural Antidote

The antidote to this dilemma is to simply compare Johnny in week one to Johnny in week two, Johnny in month one to Johnny in month two, Johnny in year one to Johnny in year two. In other words, help Johnny compete with Johnny, not with his friends. Make sure to celebrate Johnny's progress publicly (a simple high five works great), then stand back and watch his winning attitude unfold like a beautiful flower before your very eyes. With this simple strategy you'll strengthen Johnny's self confidence, constantly reignite his motivational flame, and transform the self fulfilling prophecy of failure into a self fulfilling prophecy of success.

Fulfilling Our Own Potential

Our challenge and our privilege, as professional educators, to create the conditions in which all our kids will grow stronger at everything, more confident in themselves, and more capable of taking personal responsibility for their own actions, decisions, and their own lives. To the degree we succeed, we will fulfill our own personal potentials to be *Strong at Everything, Weak at Nothing!*

An Old Coach Offers a Simple Solution to Childhood Obesity

Obesity is a huge and growing problem in America and around the world. And the childhood edition of this problem is a 21st century tragedy that's not only costing our nation billions of dollars, but it's costing millions of kids their confidence, their self esteem, their willingness to try something new in public for fear of failure, and consequently their capacity to live full and productive lives.

While scientists are busy studying body chemistry, body composition, nutrition, and exercise physiology, pharmaceutical companies are busy developing the latest weight loss pill, the diet industry is designing a new diet strategies, infomercials are crowing about new exercise devices, health clubs are hustling fitness, insurance companies are cutting benefits, and McDonald's is pushing salads, all in an effort to commercially take part in the multi billion dollar obesity industry. In the mean time, the problem continues to grow unabated, like a forest fire raging out of control.

An Old Coach's Reaction

In light of that raging forest fire I'd like to introduce you to the wisdom of a retired coach who I've known for over three decades. In the words of the old coach, "I taught physical education for most of my adult life and during that time I made the following observation. I noticed that kids who could perform pull-ups were never obese," he said. "And kids who were obese could never perform pull-ups. Pull-ups and obesity are mutually exclusive, and are never found in the same kids," he added.

Without Pills, Shots, or Magic Diets

The old coach's conclusion was that if you start 'em young, before they've had a chance to pick up much weight, teach them the ability to perform pull-ups, and teach them to never lose that ability, you can immunize kids against obesity for a lifetime, without pills, shots, magic diets, or much in the way of expense. "The more kids you can teach to physically pull their own weight," he said, "the closer you'll come to whipping the childhood obesity epidemic."

But Kids Hate Pull-Ups

I told the coach that I thought his logic was impeccable, but in my view he had one problem. According to my recollection, most kids hated pull-ups with a passion. And if they hate doing it, how can you teach them to perform pull-ups? They'll drag their feet all the way to the gym, won't they?

Using a Height Adjustable Pull-Up Bar

"Kids hate doing anything where they fail in public," the coach replied. "The trick is to start them young before they learn to associate pull-ups with public humiliation. Start them out on a height adjustable bar that allows them all to succeed immediately with leg- assisted pull-ups, jumping and pulling at the same time. With this inexpensive tool you'll eliminate failure, and build regular success into the experience for all participants."

How High Do You Set The Bar

A couple more questions popped into my mind immediately. First, how high do you set the bar when you're starting a youngster out? And secondly, how do you adjust the level of difficulty in order to insure progress? I could tell however, the wise old coach had an answer on the tip of his tongue.

The Progression

"You start the bar out low enough that the child can do at least 8 leg assisted pull-ups, but no more than 12. You allow them to work out twice a week and expect them to improve every time for a number of weeks, consecutively. In other words, in the second workout they should do 9, in the third, 10, in the fourth, 11, and in the fifth, 12 leg assisted pull-ups. When they hit 12 repetitions you raise the bar one inch and they begin the 8-12 process all over again. This strategy allows a child to make a little progress every time he or she works out, and after several weeks they learn to EXPECT TO SUCCEED IN PUBLIC, which in turn teaches them to love instead of hate pull-ups."

They've Immunized Themselves Naturally

So if I understand it right Coach, the kids literally inch their way upward until they eventually run out of leg assistance, at which point they've not only learned to perform pull-ups, but they've also learned to love doing them, and in the process they've immunized themselves naturally against obesity for a lifetime as long as they maintain the ability. Does that sound about right, I asked?

They May Want To Be Bad, But

"Mechanically speaking that's correct," the coach said. But there are a few other things that go into the strategy that you need to understand. One thing is that you're tapping into a child's natural desire to be strong and not weak. In my years of teaching I met lots of kids who wanted to be bad, but I never met a kid who wants to be weak. And that goes for the boys as well as the girls. We all want to be strong. All kids know that the ability to do pull-ups requires you to be strong. And when you work in a group, they're getting stronger in public, and kids love to succeed in public," he said. "They inevitably finish off by giving each other high fives, and they love every second of it."

I asked the coach what other things are built into his strategy. He said kids learn that three things make them strong, including regular work, good eating habits, and getting enough rest at night and in between workouts. They also learn that fooling around with tobacco, alcohol, and drugs makes them weak. And no kid ever wants to be weak. "They also learn these concepts in a very hands-on, and concrete way," he said.

Taking Responsibility For Yourself

I knew the coach could have talked on this subject all day but I wanted to finish on one other related point. The phrase "Pull Your Own Weight" has responsibility taking connotations that are very appealing to most people these days. What role does taking responsibility for oneself play in this childhood obesity prevention strategy?

After congratulating me on all the good questions the old coach said, "One of the big lessons that kids learn from working on the pull-up bar is that nobody else can do it for you," he said. "I mean in reading, writing, and arithmetic you may get away with having somebody else do your homework for awhile. But the pull-up bar knows immediately if you've done the work, it knows if you're eating right, it knows if you got enough rest recently, and it pays you for doing these things with additional success.

On the other hand, it also knows if you fail to do these things, and it can just as easily deny the public success that all kids crave. So this strategy absolutely encourages kids to take responsibility for themselves in all kinds of ways," the coach said.

A Web Site Dedicated to The Old Coach's Strategy

I confessed that he'd sold me. I agreed that teaching kids to pull their own weight would go a long ways towards solving the childhood obesity epidemic, it could save our nation billions of dollars, and do all kinds of wonderful things for the individuals who learned the lessons that are built into this simple, practical, affordable, and infinitely measurable strategy. In fact I was so impressed that I offered to build an informational web site dedicated to the old coach's naturalistic vision. He took me up on the offer, and as I write this sentence you can now check out www.pullyourownweight.net if you'd like to learn more about the old coach's simple childhood obesity prevention strategy.

One Final Question

My final question to parents and educators (or anyone who works with kids) is, why wait for the experts to come up with a high tech solution when you can turn the tide naturally with your own kids right now by simply teaching them to pull their own weight? As they always say, there's no time like the present. Carpe diem.

Strong at Everything, Weak at Nothing!

I confess, I want to be strong (i.e. independent, self-reliant, resilient) at everything and weak at nothing. And furthermore, I confess that I've never met another human being who wants to be weak at anything. In other words, every person I've ever known wants to be strong (1) at everything and weak at nothing. There are no exceptions to this rule.

Physically Strong

In my vocabulary, strong is always good, while weak is always bad, regardless of what you're talking about. For example, I want to be physically strong in order to run fast and far, jump high, move quickly from side to side, climb tall mountains, and to rescue damsels in distress. To that end my goal is to always be tangibly stronger week after week, month after month, all year long

Mentally Strong

I also want to be strong mentally. I want to be able to read great literature whether it's the Bible, the Koran, Shakespeare, Milton, Melville, Whitman, Twain, or Faulkner, and understand everything I read. I also want to be able to handle numbers like a human computer. And I want to be able to express myself clearly, concisely, insightfully, and in technicolor when and if the occasion calls for it. Yes, mental strength is a great virtue in my book.

Spiritually, Socially, Emotionally, and Psychologically Strong

I also want to be spiritually, socially, emotionally, and psychologically strong, and there's absolutely nothing at which I want to be weak. In this sense I, like all humans want to be Superman, Uberman, or God, who is by definition the alpha and the omega, the top and the bottom, the essence of essences, and obviously strong at everything and weak at nothing.

Exponentially Stronger and Stronger

But alas, as an individual human, my strength has limitations. I'm not Superman, Uberman, or God, and I never expect to be. On the other hand I've also discovered that whenever I help someone else become stronger, I can actually feel my own strength increasing week after week, month after month, all year long.

In fact when one person helps another become stronger over time, that relationship is generally considered unique. In my experience, most people don't have many of these kinds of relationships in their lives. When they have one, it stands out as something special and it's valued highly by both parties. It's the essence of a genuine parent-child, teacher-pupil, coach-player, relationship, and it's the only reason some people stay in the education field at all.

Furthermore, when I help a number of others become stronger, I find that my own strength increases even more significantly. And when those others go out and help others become stronger, my strength increases exponentially. In the midst of such a multi-level pursuit of strength, the very idea of growing stronger becomes contagious, it rubs off on others, and it spreads like a virus, a spark in a bone dry forest.

From Contagious to Radioactive

Finally, when enough people are helping enough other people grow stronger in a variety of ways, the entire atmosphere becomes super charged, super contagious, and it evolves into a stage that I like to describe as "Radioactive." Yes, when a group moves beyond contagiousness and into Radioactiveness, that's when you'll see a tipping point, a movement (i.e. civil rights, feminism), a miracle. And in the midst of this kind of miraculous experience you'll come frighteningly close to knowing yourself (and maybe even God) in the most fully human sense.

(1) The Relativity of Strength

In this book we're using the term "strength" in a relative sense. That is to say, someone who carries a heavy load needs a lot more strength than someone who carries a light load. For example, there are two people capable of doing 10 pull-ups. One of them weighs 200 lbs and the other weighs only 100 lbs. Regardless of the fact that the 200 pound fellow needs twice as much brute strength to perform the same 10 pull-ups, their relative strength is exactly the same. And if the bigger guy loses 50 pounds of excess weight, his performance and his relative strength will increase significantly even though his brute strength remains unchanged. Relative strength is all about what you can do.

The Purpose of Strength

The purpose of strength in this book is to underwrite and insure freedom, independence, self reliance, integrity, and dignity of the individual. Furthermore, it serves to avoid him/her ever becoming a burden on others, and to maximize his/her odds of being able to help others grow stronger week after week, month after month, year after year. More specifically it aims to discourage and to undermine privilege or hierarchy of any kind. This is the kind of mutually respectful strength upon which a democracy is built.

The Five Goals and Seven Habits That Make Kids Strong at Pull-ups

While working at Jefferson Elementary School in Davenport IA, we developed, organized, coordinated, and promoted a childhood obesity prevention, self esteem enhancement program called Operation Pull Your Own Weight. The program was successful in a variety of ways, and you can read about them in a variety of places.

But for the record, there were 5 specific goals, and 7 specific habits that helped kids reach their goals, along with one final challenge of which anyone aiming to duplicate this program should be aware. Without further ado, here are the 5 goals, along with the 7 habits, and the one final challenge of Operation Pull Your Own Weight.

The 5 Goals are:

1. To compete with yourself

2. To be a little stronger this week than you were last week,

3. To be a little stronger this month than you were last month,

4. And to be a lot stronger this year than you were last year.

5. Learn to do Pull-Ups

If kids accomplish these 5 goals, they'll have learned to immunize themselves against obesity for a lifetime!

The 7 Habits that make kids stronger every week, month, and year include...

1. Workout regularly

2. Eat right

3. Get enough rest

4. Avoid tobacco

5. Avoid alcohol

6. Avoid drugs

7. Take responsibility for doing these things yourself because nobody else can do them for you. It's all up to you.

The One Final Challenge:

Once the seven habits are incorporated into a kid's lifestyle, the one final challenge is to help two other kids learn to pull their own weight. Kids are inevitably amazed at how strong being able to fulfill this one final challenge makes THEM feel!

An Intriguing Side Note

And possibly the most interesting fact is that when kids apply these 5 goals, these seven habits, and this one final challenge to anything, including reading, writing, and arithmetic, they will become stronger every week, every month, and every year in those areas, and winners in the game of life.

The Seven Basic Presumptions of Operation Pull Your Own Weight

If you're an educator looking to initiate an OPYOW program at your school, your park district, your Boys and Girls Club, your YMCA/YWCA, your church, etc., these seven presumptions should be kept in mind. They represent the framework within which a successful OPYOW program is built.

1. Some kids take pride in being bad. But none take pride in being weak. We presume that all kids, regardless of gender, race, ethnicity, or economic status, want to be strong in everything. No exceptions.

2. We presume that anything perceived as a privilege (i.e. going to a movie or a ball game) is more highly valued than anything perceived as an obligation (i.e. doing your homework, cleaning your room, taking the garbage out, washing the dishes). A privilege is something you get to do, an obligation is something you have to do, and privileges are always better than obligations.

3. Being able to perform pull-ups is always associated with being relatively strong and relatively light. And if handled correctly kids can learn to value pull-ups as a privilege, an opportunity to get stronger, instead of an obligation to embarrass and humiliate themselves in front of their friends.

4. Kids who can perform pull-ups are NEVER OBESE.

5. Kids who are obese CAN NEVER PERFORM PULL-UPS.

6. Using a height adjustable pull-up bar and a technique called leg assisted pull-ups, almost any kid can learn to perform pull-ups in a predictable amount of time.

7. If it's true that kids who can do pull-ups are never obese, and almost any kid can learn to perform pull-ups, then it's irrefutably true that almost any kid can learn to immunize themselves against obesity for a lifetime by learning and maintaining the ability to perform pull-ups.

Enlightened Self Interest
and OPYOW

In one sense, the philosophical centerpiece of Operation Pull Your Own Weight is a concept known as "Enlightened Self Interest," which suggests that adults have a moral obligation to become as strong as they can, in as many ways as they can, in order to become as self sufficient as they can, and to minimize the odds of becoming dependent on others. More specifically, full fledged adults are obligated to give this self sufficiency goal no less than a 100% effort. And if they give less than 100%, they have no business expecting others to lend a helping hand when they occasionally stumble and fall.

Keeping Your Feet on Solid Ground

Inherent in the concept of *enlightened self interest* is the recognition that taking responsibility for oneself imparts a sense of dignity and self-respect on the individual who's taking that responsibility. And it's also fully understood that this dignity and self respect is one form of compensation, a great motivator that can't be expressed in dollars and cents, bought, sold or given away. In fact the only way you can get it is to earn it, which makes it a uniquely important form of compensation.

Inherent also in the concept of *enlightened self interest* is the recognition that when someone is scrambling to take care of their own affairs, it's difficult if not impossible to help anyone else take care of theirs. In other words, if you know someone who's drowning and you want to throw them a lifeline, you'd better have both feet planted solidly on dry land, or be one really strong swimmer. But if you're in the water yourself, flailing away for your own life, the odds of you helping anyone else in any way are negligible at best.

In the context of enlightened self interest, *strong is always good, and weak is always bad*. Helping someone else get stronger then is the height of virtue, a privilege, a payoff, and a return on your investment, all at the same time.

Encourages Efficiency and Discourages Excess

Enlightened self interest also recognizes that strength is a relative concept. For example, it takes twice as much upper body pulling strength for a 200 pound athlete to do 5 pull-ups as it does for a 100 pound athlete to do 5 pull-ups. As a matter of fact the relative upper body pulling strength of a100 pound athlete who can do 10 pull-ups is DOUBLE the relative strength of a 200 pound athlete who can only do 5 pull-ups. Enlightened self interest thus applauds efficiency and discourages excess of almost any kind.

From both an economic and an environmental perspective, enlightened self interest was well represented by Native American Indians who were well known for the "understanding" they had with Mother Nature. It said something like, "If we avoid taking more buffalo than we need, you will continue providing us with an abundance of buffalo." In this context nature and greed are inevitably mortal enemies. When we systematically encourage greed and arrogance, there will inevitably be a high price to pay.

Flip Sides of the Same Coin

From a linguistic perspective, enlightened self interest recognizes that in order to explain, define, and to understand self/individuality, concepts like family, group, team, and collective are necessary. After all, what is an individual self if not the opposite of a group or a team? On the other hand what is a group or a team if not a collection of individual selves?

Much like the heads and tails on a quarter flipped to start a football game, individuality and collectivity are opposite sides of the same coin. To talk in terms of the importance of one without recognizing the importance of the other is overlooking the blatantly obvious.

Enlightened VS Plain Old Self Interest

At bottom, there's a humungous difference between *enlightened self interest*, and the plain old garden variety "me first and to hexx with you" self interest, also known as selfishness, self centeredness, self righteousness, and arrogance. These are all forms of shortsightedness, if not moral ignorance and stupidity.

We're All in This Together

In contrast, enlightened self interest understands and identifies with those who say things like "What's good for my family is good for me. What's good for my neighborhood is good for my family. What's good for my city is good for my neighborhood. What's good for my county, state, nation, world, is good for my neighborhood." Arrogance lacks that kind of understanding.

Those who operate from the perspective of *enlightened self interest* also understand when someone says, "We're all in this together, so if I can help my kids get strong, that's good for me. If I can help my neighborhood get strong, that's good for my spouse and kids. If I can help my city get strong, that's good for my neighborhood, etc."

Hats off to Strong Kids

Operation Pull Your Own Weight recognizes that ALL KIDS want to be strong at everything and weak at nothing, and contends that it's the obligation of adults who work with kids (parents, teachers, etc.) to cultivate that desire, and to help all kids come as close to fulfilling their natural born strengths/potentials as possible.

Thus OPYOW suggests that individual strength is the basic building block for enlightened self interest. Without a foundation of strength and confidence, the odds of kids evolving beyond a natural and immature self centeredness to the level of enlightened self interest are bleak. Therefore, OPYOW applauds STRONG KIDS!

What Do You Expect Kids to Learn When They Participate in Operation Pull Your Own Weight?

"So Coach," they challenged, "what do you expect a student to learn when they participate in Operation Pull Your Own Weight?" That's a question I've heard repeatedly over the years, and as you might imagine, there are several answers to it.

1. The first lesson students will learn is that it's actually kind of fun and motivating to set a goal and tackle a difficult challenge like pull-ups, in front of your friends, <u>as long as you succeed</u>. Of course nobody wants to fail and embarrass themselves in front of others. But if you succeed time after time, and your friends congratulate you on each new success, you begin to expect to succeed, and to feel confident in your ability to successfully tackle a tough problem.

2. Lesson # 2 is that <u>it's a privilege</u> to be able to work with people who know how to help you become a little bit stronger (more independent) every week, every month, and every year. You see, it's the nature of all kids to want to be strong (and independent) at everything, and weak (dependent) at nothing. But not all kids get the chance to work with adults (parents or teachers) who know how to feed and cultivate that natural desire to grow stronger. But those who do will intuitively understand, and a relationship of mutual respect and appreciation will inevitably develop.

3. Lesson # 3 is that making just <u>a little slice of progress every time</u> you work out, over a long period of time, is the way you get good at anything, including pull-ups. Not only that, but making small but regular increments of progress represents a tangible return on your investment of time and effort which helps feed your motivational flame, and keeps it burning brightly over the long haul.

4. Lesson # 4 is that <u>winning is being just a little stronger</u> this week than last, a little stronger this month than last, and a lot stronger this year than last. In other words, winning is self-mastery and it has almost nothing to do with others. Compete with yourself day after day, week after week, month after month, year after year, and you'll have nothing to fear from others.

5. Lesson # 5 is that <u>there are seven habits</u> that make you strong on the pull-up bar (and everything else) including regular practice, eating right, getting sufficient rest, avoiding tobacco, alcohol, and drugs, and taking responsibility for doing these things yourself because nobody else can do them for you.

6. Lesson # 6 is that if you learn to do pull-ups and maintain the ability, you will always be <u>relatively strong and physically efficient</u> (trim). And if you apply these principals to all other aspects of your life you'll not only become physically efficient, but mentally and spiritually efficient as well. In doing so you will successfully climb your own personal Mt. Potential and you'll live your life on the level at which it was meant to be lived.

7. Lesson # 7 is that once you've learned to master the activity yourself, one of the most fulfilling and gratifying experiences you can ever have is to <u>help someone else</u> learn and master these same strength building habits. In other words, helping someone else discover their own strength and confidence multiplies your own strength and confidence exponentially, and that's incredibly fulfilling.

Imbedded Into Your DNA

Practiced regularly, week after week, month after month, year after year, these hands-on, eyeball to eyeball, ultimately practical lessons become habitual, second nature, imbedded into your subconscious, your DNA. They become the eyes through which you view the world. And that's strength you can count on.

Privilege VS Obligation
When Pulling Your Own Weight

As he reached the last rung on the monkey bars, his face grimacing, his little hands grabbing hold and hanging on tight, Billy Jr. dropped to the ground, beamed with pride, and crowed, "Dad, did you see that? I made it all the way to the end!"

Bill Sr. smiled broadly at his son and gave him a high five. "You're really getting strong aren't you Billy," his dad said with a tangible sense of pride in his own voice.

Kids Naturally Revel In Physical Achievement

Now with this picture in mind, you'll know what I mean when I say that *kids naturally enjoy, even revel in their physical achievements* starting with the first finger they grab, and the first step they take. And just because a task is difficult and challenging doesn't mean that it's any less enjoyable for kids. As long as the goal is valued, (i.e. reaching the last rung on the monkey bars) difficulty even increases the enjoyment.

Kids Are Naturally Curious and Creative

Kids are not naturally lazy and slothful. On the contrary, they're natural born explorers of their environments. They're curious about everything and everyone around them. When they see it, they naturally want to reach out and touch it, grab it, taste it, smell it, hear it, and experience it as fully as possible. That's how and why kids grow so quickly in their formative years.

Privilege VS Obligation

Since kids are naturally programmed to explore themselves and the world around them, *the challenge for a legitimate educator* is to tap into that natural curiosity, to cultivate it, to encourage it, to grow it, day after day, week after week, month after month. But in order for that to happen, education must be presented and perceived as something the child gets to do, not something the child has to do. In other words, education must be seen as a privilege, an opportunity, instead of an obligation, a job.

Keeping The Flame Lit...

When this challenge is met, and this goal is achieved, the child's natural sense of curiosity will remain inflamed, and they will continue to soak in new knowledge from new experiences, and they'll also come to understand and appreciate the fulfillment that learning, in the best sense, has to offer.

Or Extinguishing It

On the contrary, when we inadvertently turn education into a job, complete with commutes, daily starting times, tasks that have to be completed whether the child wants to do them or not, and extrinsic rewards (i.e. stars and grades) that transform the natural born learner into an object to be compared and judged against others, the flame is extinguished. The child quickly learns that what adults call education is not fun, is not something you get to do, is not a privilege, but a job, an obligation, and something to avoid whenever possible. Kids and teachers live for the weekend, and summer vacation.

Regular Improvement Feeds The Flame

For these reasons, it's essential for anyone wanting to teach a child to physically *Pull Their Own Weight*, that pull-ups be presented and perceived as something the child gets to do, not something they have to do. And the key to growing that curiosity flame and that privileged status lies in making sure the child walks away from each experience feeling successful, feeling better this time than last time, feeling as if there was a payoff for the time and effort invested. We'll explore that topic next.

Bad But Never Weak...

Remember, lots of kids today want to be bad. But you'll never meet a kid who wants to be weak. They all want to be strong at everything and weak at nothing.

Documented Results...
The Missing Ingredient in Childhood Obesity Prevention

After shaking hands with the old coach (he prefers to avoid being mentioned by name) who I've known now for over 30 years, we walked into the gym and he started pointing out kids to me. "See Tommy over there standing by the door? He's improved from 3 to 9 pull-ups in the past four months," the coach said. "Tommy knows that *as long as he can do those pull-ups, he'll always be strong*, which is why he keeps working on getting better," the coach said.

Tommy, the First Documented Result

Tommy is just one example of the DOCUMENTED RESULTS part of the coach's obesity prevention program appropriately called Operation Pull Your Own Weight. He continued by pointing to a girl named Suzette who was playing one on one basketball against a boy named Joey. As the coach explained, Suzette has yet to master conventional pull-ups, but she's been working hard on reaching that goal.

Suzette, the Second Documented Result

"Suzette's working out three times a week on a height adjustable pull-up bar, using leg assisted pull-ups in order to teach herself to do pull-ups," the coach said. "She's also keeping a chart that shows exactly what she's accomplished, workout to workout over the past couple of months. Actually she can come pretty close to predicting when she'll reach her goal. And *every step of it is documented* in black and white," he added.

The Essence of OPYOW

The Operation Pull Your Own Weight program is based on three simple observations. The first is that kids who can do pull-ups *are never much overweight*. The second is that, using a height adjustable pull-up bar in conjunction with leg assisted pull-ups (jumping and pulling at the same time), *almost all kids can learn to do pull-ups*. And third, if almost all kids can learn to do pull-ups,

34

then *almost all kids can immunize themselves against obesity for a lifetime* by learning to do pull-ups, and maintaining the ability for the rest of their lives.

Wall A, Wall B

In the coach's own words, "Walk into any gym class in America and ask those kids who can do at least one pull-up to stand by wall A, and ask those who can't to stand by wall B. What you'll see is what I like to call the great fitness divide, where the kids on wall A are relatively strong and light, and the kids on wall B are relatively weak and/or heavy. Our strategy is to move as many kids as possible from wall B to wall A and to celebrate their immunization against obesity. Tommy is a member of wall A and Suzette will be soon. *And both can document their success week to week, month to month.*

Most Obesity Prevention Programs Lack Documented Results

So, documented results seemed to occupy center stage for the coach's OPYOW program. "Without documented success," he said, "no program can justify its existence. That's the main problem with 99% of the obesity prevention programs being promoted across the nation. The government and many others have spent billions over the past decade, and the only thing they have to show for it is boatloads of failure."

I Challenge You to Prove Me Wrong

"We're losing the war on childhood obesity, and all the experts with all their degrees are wringing their hands over trying to get a handle on the problem. They don't have a single Tommy who's effectively immunized himself against obesity for a lifetime as long as he can do pull-ups. They don't have one Suzette who can show you a weekly report on the progress she's making towards eliminating the possibility of obesity in her life. Those are just two of many documented success stories we have in this school and I challenge anyone to prove me wrong," the coach said.

Let's Get Some Detail

So I asked the coach to talk more about OPYOW's documented results and to explain them in a little more detail. He of course obliged. "If you can show any of these kids that there's a tangible return on their investment of time and effort, and that *they're making consistent, documented progress towards a valued goal, they'll motivate themselves to get the job done*. Not only that," the coach said, "but their enthusiasm is contagious and it rubs off on friends. Pretty soon you'll have a bunch of kids who are excited over immunizing themselves against obesity for a lifetime because I guarantee you, not one of them has ever wanted to be obese."

They Won't Sacrifice Their Cool
"On the other hand," he continued, "if you put these kids in a position where they're likely to fail in front of their friends, you put them in a position where they have to choose between risking failure and humiliation, or maintaining their cool by just refusing to try. Give them that choice and *a high percentage will stop trying* and shoot themselves in the foot before they risk being uncool."

Small Bites Plus Relentless Persistence
"We go to great lengths to avoid putting our kids in that predicament. We teach that success occurs in small bites, and when combined with relentless persistence over weeks, months, and years, those small bites add up to large chunks of success. In other words we teach kids to experience success, and to expect success. And to OPYOW, success is when you're just a little bit better this time than you were last time, every week, every month, all year long," the coach said.

Motivation That Fees on Itself
"And as long as our students really expect to succeed, they'll be motivated, and they'll persist, relentlessly, until they achieve the goals they've set for themselves. In this case they'll immunize themselves against obesity for a lifetime. If they expect to fail though, there's no reason to try. When they stop trying they're automatically destined to fail. Failure becomes the proverbial self fulfilling prophecy."

Reading, Writing, and Arithmetic
"By the way, this same formula works for anything including reading, writing, and arithmetic. Take documented results and

36

success out of the formula though, and you're back at square one, scratching your head. It's all about being able to deliver documented results," he said with a smile.

P.S. How About Requiring Pull-ups for Graduation

Just then an interesting thought struck me. What if we made the ability to do pull-ups a graduation requirement? I said it out loud to the old coach and he thought for a second.

Then he said, "I've had similar thoughts myself, but making pull-ups a graduation requirement turns them into an obligation instead of an opportunity, and in the process you'd blow a big hole in the motivational balloon. I'd rather see students learn it on their own because they want to do it, instead of on the orders of anyone. That's an interesting thought though I must admit," he added.

The Many Virtues of
Infinite Measurability

One of the major stumbling blocks in defeating childhood obesity is the lack of measurability, a way to conveniently evaluate progress, which results in a lack of motivation, and an epidemic that continues to grow like a forest fire raging out of control.

As a matter of fact the National Institute of Medicine recently issued a disturbing report indicating that after spending over $68,000,000 over five years on just one program (there were many others), because of poor evaluation methods, we still have no idea what works and what doesn't work. We wasted $68,000,000. Imagine that.

If You Can't Measure It, How Do You Know

But if you lack the ability to measure accurately how will you ever know if you're winning, losing, or just spinning your wheels? The State of Arkansas for example, is considered to be one of the nation's leaders in the battle against childhood obesity. Bill Clinton has even gotten into the fray. They decided to measure every child's body mass index (the most commonly used indicator) and put it on their report card once every quarter…in other words, every nine weeks.

How Do You Motivate Kids

But even if this measurement is accurate and meaningful for kids, which is highly questionable in itself, getting feedback once every nine weeks packs almost no motivational punch at all. By the same token it's economically impractical to measure on a daily, weekly, or even monthly basis. Once a quarter is about the best they can do.

Other more sophisticated measurement possibilities such as testing percentage of body fat via electronic impedance (computer) or underwater weighing are dramatically more expensive and much less likely to be used by anyone except a professor or grad student in a physiology lab. Furthermore, such models focus on the negative…how fat are you instead of how strong are you? A lack of regular feedback, in combination with their negative connotations

DOOM the most conventional strategies to failure. And after years of work, and multi millions spent, we still don't know what works and what doesn't work.

Kindergartner Can Measure This

In contrast, the documented measurability factor in a program called Operation Pull Your Own Weight is extremely regular, and highly practical. You need no special instruments, no magic formulas, and almost no specialized training to tell if students are improving or not. If you can count from one to twelve, as most kindergartners can, you qualify. As a matter of fact, elementary school age kids not only can, but they have measured themselves and others without problem. Not only that, but the strength gain focus of this program has very positive, not negative connotations.

The Feedback is Constant

More specifically, OPYOW is based on the old coach's observation that kids who can do pull-ups can't be obese. And kids who are obese can't do pull-ups. The ability to do pull-ups and obesity are mutually exclusive and where you find one, you'll not find the other.

Now, using a height adjustable pull-up bar and leg assisted pull-ups, (the child's encouraged to jump and pull at the same time) most kids can learn to do pull-ups. The idea is to count and record (document change) the number of repetitions a participant can perform at a particular bar height. The program is initiated by finding a bar height at which a participant can do eight leg assisted pull-ups which constitutes workout # one. In workout # 2 they do nine, in workout # 3 they do ten, in workout # 4 they do eleven, and in workout # 5 they do twelve leg assisted pull-ups. Then in workout # 6 the bar is raised one inch and the whole eight to twelve scenario begins all over again.

The Motivation is High

In other words each participant is taught how to improve regularly, in very small increments every week, every month, over a prescribed period of time. The progress is highly visible, highly motivating, INFINITELY MEASURABLE, and the positive feedback occurs every single time the participant works out.

Under these conditions, along with public success and celebration (high fives), motivation remains high throughout the program, evaluation becomes extremely easy and affordable, and the focus on strength gain instead of fat loss is positive not negative. In other words, Operation Pull Your Own Weight is extremely affordable, extremely motivating, and INFINITELY MEASURABLE, DOCUMENTABLE, AND EVALUATEABLE.

And In The End, You'll Know

At the end of a week, a month, a quarter, a year, you'll know, unequivocally, if you're winning the war, losing the war, or just treading water. You'll never be in a position where you've just spent $68,000,000 and are still groping in the dark for answers. Not only that, but you'll defeat childhood obesity naturally, without resorting to pills, shots, and special diets to get the job done.

Mother Nature Defines Fitness In Functional, Not Cosmetic Terms

In nature, out in the wild, animals who are overweight (unfit) are not tolerated, and obesity just can't happen. If an antelope for example, gains a few extra pounds, he gets one step slower and becomes easy prey for Mamma lion. If Mamma lion picks up a few extra pounds, she won't catch up to the antelope. As the result she'll naturally miss a few meals, eventually sheds the excess weight, and she'll be back in the hunt.

Moving a little closer to home, if a squirrel picks up extra weight, he'll be unable to climb trees or leap from limb to limb with total abandon. He may even miss, fall, and become a tasty treat for the local Jack Russell Terrier. And if a robin in your backyard picks up a little extra luggage, she'll have a harder time getting off the ground and into flight. At that point a local cat might just make a meal out of her.

I could go on and on here, but I'm sure you see the point that, out in the wild (even the suburban wilderness), where survival depends on an animal's ability to avoid a predator, or a predator's ability to catch up to its prey, there's simply zero tolerance for excess body weight if an animal wants to continue breathing.

The Lone Exception to Mother Nature's Ironclad Rule

The only instance where Mother Nature temporarily tolerates excess weight is with animals that hibernate for a certain period of the year. The bear for example, is an animal who, before going into hibernation takes on extra calories, packs on an extra layer of fat, goes to sleep for several months, intending to eat nothing. He's effectively living off of the stored fat in his system.

But when the bear awakes in the spring, the excess weight will be gone, and he's back in the position of having to earn his daily meals by catching up with his prey every day, and his excess weight will be gone for the season.

Obesity and Domestication

Other than that, excess weight is found only in domesticated animals. That is to say you'll find fat pigs, and hefty heifers out on the farm. You'll see fat dogs and occasionally even fat cats who have become so domesticated and dependent on their human masters that they've fattened up to the point of being physically incapable of surviving in the wild. Animals that don't have to physically earn their daily bread, or physically avoid being turned into someone else's daily bread, have the option of becoming overweight. But any animal that has to catch his prey, or run from a predator, can ill afford the luxury of being overweight.

And What About Our Closest Ancestor?

Before moving on to the domesticated human species let's take a quick look at man's closest cousin, the monkey (or the gorilla). In fact let me ask, can you even imagine seeing a fat monkey or gorilla out in the wild? If a monkey gains much weight, climbing trees with the greatest of ease, and swinging from limb to limb Tarzan style, becomes a physical impossibility. The result? No fat monkeys in the jungle!

What Can We Learn From Mother Nature?

So Mother Nature basically defines fitness (or the lack of it) in functional terms, not in cosmetic terms. That is to say, she wants to know what you can do with your body, not what do you look like. On the other hand it's also no secret that there's a definite sense of beauty found in a well developed, fully functioning, and confident human physique, and in many cultures, including the ancient Greeks. They celebrated it.

But in nature it's function first and beauty second, not the other way around. With all that said, let's ask what can modern, domesticated man learn from Mother Nature, and how can we apply this knowledge to the childhood obesity epidemic sitting out on our front doorstep? Let's talk about that right now.

The Peace Corps' Solution To Obesity

In light of our previous comments about Mother Nature and her intolerance for obesity at almost any level, one solution to the obesity problem would be to chuck the modern lifestyle that encourages poor eating habits and inactivity, and go back into the wild. It's not as if that has not been done before. Certain kinds of scientists do it on a regular basis in order to study nature in various ways.

I have a good friend who volunteered for the Peace Corps and served a year in Africa (Gambia to be precise) and he confirmed that overeating and lack of physical exercise are non-existent in the Gambian tribal cultures where he lived for a year. This guy, by the way was trim when he left, and even trimmer when he came back. There are also missionaries who represent various church groups who go into the third world, and who actually benefit physically from the lack of junk food and television sets.

Answer This Simple Question

But presuming that you're not an Indiana Jones kind of scientist, or that you're not the missionary type, and the Peace Corps just doesn't fit into the schedule right now, what are your naturalistic options here in domestic captivity? In order to best answer that question let me pose another question. How many activities can you make the following statement about? I CAN'T BE OVERWEIGHT AS LONG AS I CAN STILL DO

_____! Use your imagination and see what you can come up with.

Three Easy To See Examples...

There are lots of answers to that question. How about running fast or running long? I mean, people who are overweight can't run fast or long right? Let's test the statement and see if it makes sense. I can't be overweight as long as I can still run fast or run long. Does that work for you? It sure does for me. Let's try another one.

How about jumping high or long? I know people who can get way off the floor on a vertical jump test. These same people can jump lengthwise as well. But those who can perform these feats are definitely not overweight. So here we go again...I can't be overweight as long as I can still jump high or jump long. Another winner, right?

Let's try one more to make sure we have it straight. How about climbing on climbing walls, or on the sides of mountains? I've seen lots of photos of climbers and I've never seen one who's carrying any excess weight. So, I can't be overweight as long as I can still climb the wall or the mountain. That's one more in the winner's circle, right?

So what kinds of conclusions can we draw from these observations that are pertinent to the childhood obesity issue? Would you agree with me if I said "if a child learns to run fast or long, climb a wall or the side of a mountain, or jump high or long, you can safely bet on the fact that they will not be overweight?" It's really quite simple. Where you have functional ability, whether it's in the wilds of darkest Africa or in the suburbs of Chicago, you will find no instances of overweight/obesity.

But My Kid's A Musician Not An Athlete...

But you say "Wait a minute. What if I live in the city and my children don't have the time, the opportunity, or the desire to learn to run, jump, or climb? What if my kids are more into music or drama or academics? Aren't there any naturalistic, functional options for them to choose from?" The answer is...there sure are. Let's have a look.

Dips On The Parallel Or Monkey Bars

Dips are an exercise performed on parallel bars or monkey bars in which the participant starts in the up position, lowers him/herself down into the down position, and then pushes him/herself back up again. The exercise works the chest and the triceps primarily, and it's most often seen in gymnastic oriented activities. Dips are an exercise in which the entire body weight is the resistance factor and if you can do any of them the odds of being overweight are very minimal.

Dips, like all body weight exercises, pay for fat loss and for strength (muscle) gain. That means that if you improve your ability to do dips, you're either losing fat, gaining muscle, or both. Which is just another way of saying your body composition is improving and your percentage of body fat is going down. So let's give dips our little test right now. I can't be overweight if I can still do dips. This one works for me.

Hand Stand Push Ups

Another good example is an exercise known as handstand push ups. As the name indicates, in this exercise you flip upside

44

down and stand on your hands instead of your feet, and balance yourself. Then you lower yourself down, touch your nose to the floor, and push yourself back up into the starting position.

The one factor that comes into play for this exercise is balance. You can be strong and lean, and have a poor sense of balance which undermines your ability to perform hand stand push ups. But other than that, the scenario works. This exercise pays for any performer to lose fat, gain strength, for body composition improvement, and a reduction in percentage of body fat. Shall we try our test? I can't be overweight as long as I can still do hand stand push ups. Absolutely true, right? It works once again.

Superman Push Ups

The third example I'd like to talk about is called the Superman Push Up, because when the participant is doing the exercise they look like Superman flying over Metropolis looking for Lex Luthor or some other super villain doing bad things to good people. All that aside, the participant performs this exercise with an exercise wheel in hand, starting in what is the conventional push up position. They roll the wheel out until they're stretched out in the Superman position, and then roll back up into the starting position.

This exercise is very challenging to the core muscles (the abdominals and the lower back) and if done wrong it can cause lower back problems. However it definitely pays the participant to lose fat, gain strength, improve body composition, and reduce your percentage of body fat. As for the test, let's give it a try. If I can still do Superman Push Ups, I can't be overweight. Yep, that works again, doesn't it?

Sissy Squats

Sissy squats are basically leg extensions that use the participant's own body weight as the resistance. Blocking off the front of the ankles and the back of the knees, you lower yourself backwards until your thighs are parallel with the ground. If you bend at the waist this exercise is much easier than if you remain straight from the knees up…in other words if you avoid bending at the waist.

Sissy squats isolate the quadriceps and they pay for fat loss, strength gain, improved body composition, and reduced percentage

45

of body fat. In other words sissy squats are not really for sissies, and if I can still do the most difficult variety of sissy squats, I can't be overweight? That's absolutely true.

Rope Climbing

The fourth example I want to talk about is Rope Climbing. If you're in school you may have seen this done in the recent past. If you're out of school you may have to recollect your days in gym class. Either way, if you can start at the bottom, climb to the top, and let yourself back down under control (avoiding a roper burn, which is the potential negative factor with this one), that's a pretty darn good trick.

The rope pays for fat loss, strength gain, improved body composition, and reduced percentage of body fat. And I can't be overweight as long as I can still climb a rope. The statement is absolutely true then about rope climbing, sissy squats, Superman push ups, hand stand push ups, and dips. If you can do any one of them, and maintain the ability, you are not now, and you never will be overweight. Now there's an interesting thought in the midst of an obesity epidemic, wouldn't you agree?

Any <u>One</u> of These Will Work For Any Body

I'm here to say that *any one of these exercises, alone and by themselves, could serve as a functional antidote to childhood obesity*, adolescent obesity, and adult obesity without a pill, without a health club membership, without a degree in Physical Education, and with hardly any time or expense to speak of. It's perfect for students who are into music, debate, art, and drama instead of sports and athletics. And they're all natural, something that Mother Nature might expect of her own animal population out in the wild.

And Then There Are Pull-ups

Are there any other exercises that would immunize and vaccinate any human being, including all children, against being overweight? You could discover more if you really put your mind to it. But there's one more in particular that I want to mention because for my money it's the best example. But you're going to have to move on to the next chapter to discover everything I want to tell you about a wonderful little exercise called PULL-UPS.

The Mechanics of

Operation Pull Your Own Weight

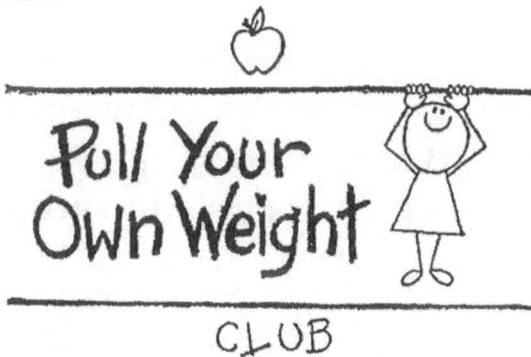

Leg Assisted Pull-ups on Height Adjustable Pull-up Straps
(The Nuts and Bolts of OPYOW)

1. Attach straps/grips to any pull-up bar in any gym.

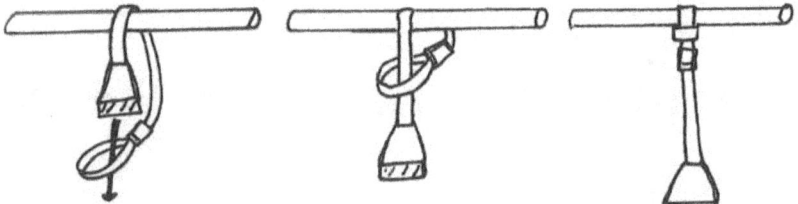

1. Place handle over pull up bar

2. Thread handle and strap through attachment loop.

3. Pull tight to secure straps.

2. Adjust the grip's height to a level where the student feet are on the floor and they can EASILY perform 8 leg assisted pull-ups (jumping/pulling simultaneously).

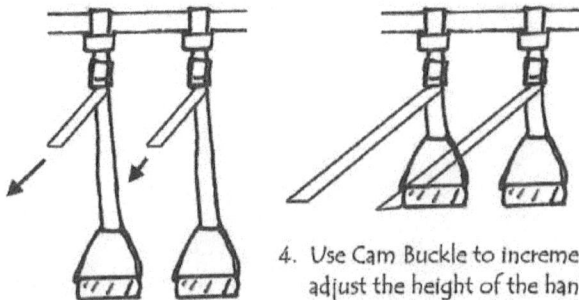

4. Use Cam Buckle to incrementaly adjust the height of the handles

3. Allow the student to perform 8 leg assisted pull-ups (all the way up - chin touching the grips, and all the way down - feet touching the floor), and designate as workout # 1.

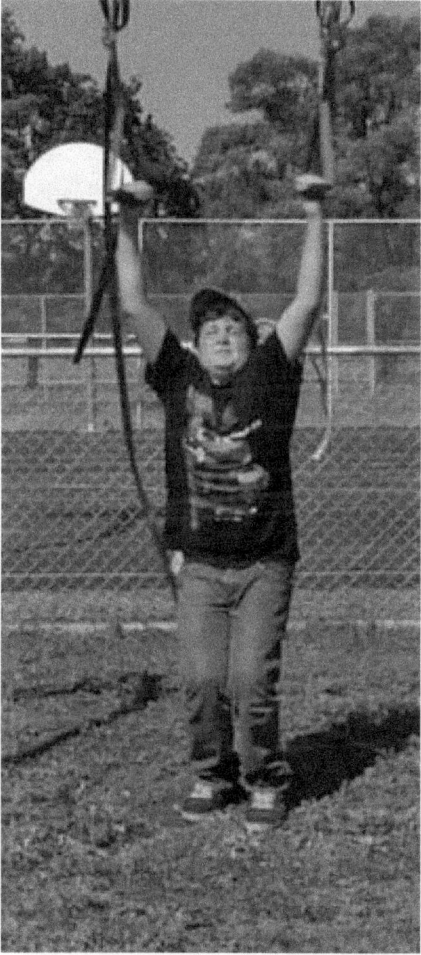

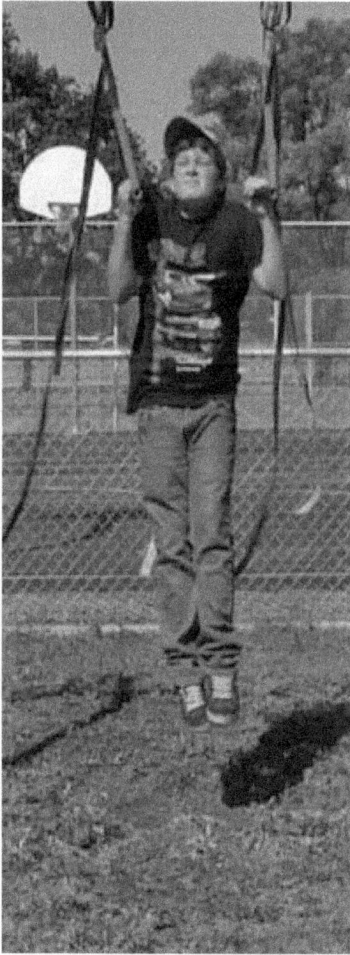

4. DOCUMENT it on the OPYOW Progress Chart

OPYOW 10 Week Sample Progress Chart

Name _____

Start Date_____

Date	Level (in Inches)	Reps

REMEMBER...

2 Workouts Per Week

AND YOUR GOALS ARE TO BECOME:
- **A Little Stronger This Week Than Last!**
- **A Little Stronger This Month Than Last!**
- **A Lot Stronger This Year Than Last!**

5. We suggest students should do 2 workouts per week, on NON-CONSECUTIVE days, i.e. Mon/Thurs, Tues/Fri).

6. Workout # 2 the student performs 9 leg assisted pull-ups

7. Workout # 3 the student performs 10 leg assisted pull-ups

8. Workout # 4 the student performs 11 leg assisted pull-ups

9. Workout # 5 the student performs 12 leg assisted pull-ups

10. DOCUMENT each and every workout on the student's OPYOW Progress Chart.

11. In Workout # 6 THE GRIPS ARE RAISED ONE INCH, and the entire 8 to 12 routine is repeated all over again for five more consecutive workouts.

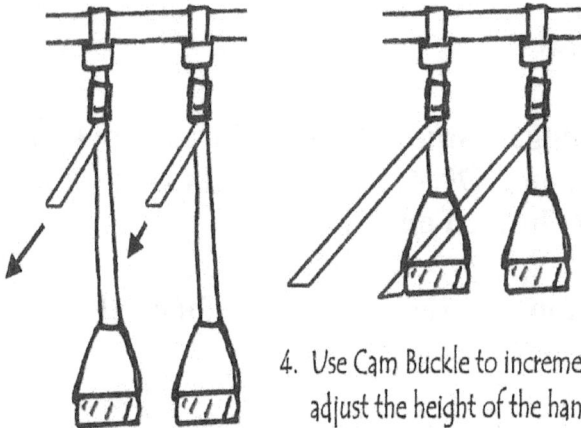

4. Use Cam Buckle to incrementaly adjust the height of the handles

12. So for example, every 2.5 weeks (5 workouts) the grips are raised one inch. That means in 10 weeks, the grips will have been raised FOUR INCHES, and the student will have experienced <u>documented progress in 20 consecutive workouts</u> in front of their peers, along with the high fives, and confidence that accompanies it. They will also learn to look forward to each new opportunity to get on the grips (bar) and to get stronger, in front of their friends, because succeeding in public is FUN! Success, breeds success.

13. Experiencing very small, but consistent increments of progress, over an extended period of time encourages high levels of motivation, which translates into persistence. Eventually the student will run out of leg assistance, at which point they're able to do conventional pull-ups and will have naturally immunized themselves against obesity for life, as long as they maintain the ability to do pull-ups.

14. The only thing left now is to START NOW! Procrastination is the opposite of ACTION!

Childhood Obesity Prevention and Functional Body Composition Testing

School A uses Body Mass Index (BMI) to determine which students are obese and which ones are not. School B uses the skin fold method (calipers measuring skin thickness), School C uses electronic impedance (a computerized method), while School D does under water weighing at the local University Physiology lab to determine their student's body composition (usually expressed as a percentage of body fat).

Conventional VS Functional

In other words schools A, B, C, and D use conventional forms of measurement and data to determine how physically efficient their students are, and to predict how well they will perform in various arenas, including the physical/athletic arena. School E however, takes precisely the opposite approach by measuring physical performance and using that data to determine how physically efficient their students are, and to predict what their percentages of body fat will be.

When One Goes Up, the Other Goes Down

"It's pretty simple" said Coach E. "When percentage of body fat goes down, performance goes up. And when percentage of body fat goes up, performance goes down. These two factors are directly related to one another, and when one of them changes, the other reflects those changes simultaneously."

In the end, what everyone's really aiming for is to improve performance in all arenas. So why even fool around with BMI's, skin calipers, electronic impedance devices, and underwater weighing when performance can be measured directly, yielding everything anyone needs to know about a student's physical efficiency?

For Example: Instead of Conventional Measurements

In place of all the conventional measurements for example, Coach E uses a pull-up bar. (1) More specifically he uses a height adjustable pull-up bar in conjunction with a technique called leg assisted pull-ups that allows students to keep their feet on the floor, jump and pull at the same time. This strategy gives all his students immediate access, a viable starting point when learning to perform pull-ups.

Progress, Motivation, and Persistence

Progress is achieved in very small increments (i.e. one more repetition, or raising the bar one inch). Small increments encourage regular progress, instill motivation, and cultivate a sense of RELENTLESS PERSISTENCE until conventional pull-ups are finally mastered.

Immunized Against Obesity for Life

"Under these conditions" Coach E said, "our kid's performances improve regularly. And along with performance improvement comes an improvement in body composition. The basic goal of our program is to help each student learn to perform conventional pull-ups, because, as any PE teacher will tell you, kids who can do pull-ups are NEVER OBESE. And as long as they maintain their ability to perform pull-ups, these kids are naturally immunized against obesity for life. How's that for a mega-payoff?"

Increased Performance Equals Improved Body Composition

At the next level, once they can perform conventional pull-ups, any increase in performance indicates an improved body composition, and vice-versa. For example, if a student's pull-up performance goes from 10 to 20, they've either gained muscle/strength, lost fat, or both, so their body composition has improved. On the other hand, if the student's pull-up performance goes from 20 to 10, they've either lost muscle/strength, gained fat, or both, so their body composition has deteriorated along with their performance.

Victory Over Childhood Obesity

In the long run, the goal of Coach E's program is to graduate an entire class full of students who are all functionally immunized against obesity for life because they can all perform pull-ups. "When that day arrives," Coach E said, "We'll declare victory over childhood obesity in our school. Until then, we'll keep making DOCUMENTED PROGRESS one repetition at a time, one inch at a time, and one child at a time, and leave all the conventional measurement devices to the experts," coach E added.

(1) Pull-ups are not the only exercise capable of making this claim. Other challenging body weight exercises such as dips, rope climbing, sissy squats, and vertical jumping will yield all the same insightful information regarding body composition/physical efficiency issues.

Functional Fitness and Functional Beauty

The term functional fitness comes from the world of athletics where the coach doesn't really care what you look like in a photograph or the mirror. Instead he cares about how fast you can run, how high you can jump, how far and how fast can you throw, how hard and how often can you hit, and how accurately can you shoot, etc.?

You can resemble the Frankenstein monster himself, but if you can perform these previously mentioned tasks with great efficiency, power, endurance, flexibility, fluidity, and coordination you'll look astonishingly beautiful to any coach. But to be fair to the coach, there's something inherently attractive, and yes beautiful about the human body in motion. Just ask the ancient Greeks who turned the likes of a human discus thrower into great art, including sculptures that we still admire in the 21st century.

Air Jordan Mid-Air

But if we turn the page to the modern era, think of the silhouetted Michael Jordan launching himself from the top of the free throw circle, ball in one hand, en route to slam dunking a basketball. Think of Bear greats Gayle Sayers and Devon Hester bobbing and weaving their way through 11 defenders bent on their immediate destruction. Think of Jumpin' Joe Dimmagio swinging his classic baseball bat, Jesse Owens sprinting or long jumping in Nazi Germany, Muhammad Ali demolishing Sonny Listen or George Foreman and you will recognize that there is a distinct sense of beauty in the powerful and efficient movements of the human body itself.

Opposed to Excess and Complication

In other words, in the world of functional fitness you don't need a movie star's face to be considered beautiful. In the world of functional fitness you don't need Mary Kay, Maybeline, Revlon, Rolex, Ralph Lauren, ear rings, or mega muscles to cause a viewer to stand awestruck over the beauty of the human body in motion. In the world of functional beauty it's all about the human body in motion doing what it is capable of doing with maximum efficiency and flow whether running, jumping, throwing, catching, swinging, hitting, climbing, shooting, diving, pushing, pulling, twirling, or dancing.

Self Confidence of Functional Fitness

And along with functional fitness comes a unique, inner form of self confidence and self respect that's not for sale at the cosmetic counter or the local pharmacy, on the latest television infomercial, or even over the vast Internet. Functional fitness is 33% earned, 33% genetic, and 33% inherited opportunity. But it's never 100% purchased. Functional fitness and functional beauty are essentially simple, natural, lean, efficient, and opposed to excess in any form. They're also fast, quick, flexible, balanced, coordinated, rhythmic, powerful, purposeful, and fully capable of enduring.

How Do You Get It?

So how do you get it? There's an age old adage that says "form follows function." In other words, what you do heavily influences or even dictates what you look like. So for example if you do a lot of long distance running your body will eventually begin to take on the form of a lean long distance runner. If you do a lot of swimming your body will eventually begin to take on the form of a swimmer's body. If you pump a lot of iron, do a lot of gymnastics, play a lot of tennis, take up ball room dancing, tai chi, or sitting in front of a computer eight hours a day week in and week out, those choices will be reflected in the form of your physical presence, your body.

A Form of Beauty to Be Reckoned With

Form follows function. Function precedes form. Functional fitness is essentially dynamic not static, and is a form of beauty to be recognized and to be reckoned with.

Functional Performance Instead of Underwater Weighing, Electronic Impedance, Skin Calipers, or BMI

The car is fully packed and the family is ready for vacation. And when I say fully packed, I mean that 800 pounds of luggage is stuffed into the trunk, as well as in and around the kids in the back seat. You can hardly see out of the rear view mirror because you've packed so much into this poor car.

You drive down the highway for the first 100 miles and notice that your car's normal pick up seems to be lacking, and the fuel gauge is dropping faster than usual, so you pull off the road and decide to try something drastic. One by one you take each piece of luggage out of the trunk, and the back seat of the car, and place them all carefully alongside the road. I mean you eliminate everything but the wife and kids. Then you proceed to put the car in gear and drive on down the road.

Suddenly you notice that your car's pick up and the gas gauge are both back to normal. In other words the physical performance of your car has suddenly improved now that you've eliminated all the excess weight. In engineering terms this phenomena is commonly known as improving your car's "Power to Weight Ratio."

Cars, Planes, and Human Bodies

The power to weight principle applies whether you're throwing excess weight out of your car or out of an airplane. Maintain the horsepower, eliminate non-functional, excess weight, and performance automatically improves. Interestingly enough, it applies just as well to the human body. Hang on to your horsepower (your muscle/strength), eliminate the excess weight (fat) and like magic, your physical performance automatically improves (and vice versa).

A Direct Relationship

But what I'd like to focus on here is the direct relationship between your physical efficiency and your functional performance.

That is to say, when your physical efficiency (your percentage of body fat) improves, your functional performance (i.e. running, jumping, climbing) automatically improves. When your physical efficiency (your percentage of body fat) deteriorates, your performance automatically deteriorates.

Let's Get Practical About Measuring Body Composition

That being the case, I'd like to pose the following question. If physical efficiency (body composition) is automatically reflected in functional performance, why does anyone need to measure anyone's percentage of body fat with under water weighing, electronic impedance, or with skin calipers? Furthermore, if physical efficiency is automatically reflected in functional performance, why would anyone ever bother measuring anyone's BMI?

It seems to me that the aim of improving anyone's percentage of body fat, their body composition, or their physical efficiency (these are all the same thing) is to improve their functional performance. And if you improve their functional performance, you're automatically improving their physical efficiency as well as their percentage of body fat, and their body composition.

Choose One Functional Activity and Master It

So why not just choose one functional activity (i.e. pull-ups, dips, or rope jumping), get a base line, train to improve that one activity, day after day, week after week, month after month, and recognize that the participant's physical efficiency, their percentage of body fat, and their body composition are all improving automatically, simultaneously?

Why even waste anyone's time with underwater weighing, electronic impedance, skin fold measurements, or BMI, when all of these are directly and automatically reflected in functional performance changes? To eliminate obesity simply choose one functional activity (pull-ups, dips, or rope climbing), practice it week after week, month after month, master it, and maintain the mastery. When mastery is maintained, obesity (physical inefficiency) becomes impossible.

Coach, I Can't Do Pull-ups: What Now?

"So Coach," my colleague said. "What happens if I run into students who are genetically predisposed to being unable to do conventional pull-ups? What should I do with them?"

My first answer was to point out that, if you start them young, like kindergarten, first and second grade, there are very few kids who are unable to learn to do conventional pull-ups. You just have to give them a place to start, a way to make regular progress on their way to developing the ability to do their own edition of conventional pull-ups.

Exceptions to Every Rule

On the other hand, I won't go so far as to claim there are no exceptions. There are always exceptions to any rule, and for those exceptions, here's what I suggest.

If you start them young on leg assisted pull-ups, with the bar so low that their chin is even with the bar while their feet are still flat on the floor, allow no jumping, keep the height constant, and simply increase the reps (down and up, over and over again) from week to week, month to month, these kids will make regular, documented progress towards eliminating obesity in their lives, even if they never learn to do conventional pull-ups.

For Example

Here's how it goes. Find a starting point where the number of reps are easy for these kids to do. It could be 3, 5, 7, or 20 leg assisted pull-ups. I repeat it should be EASY for them. How easy you ask? It should be so easy that the student is absolutely certain that he or she can do one more rep in their next workout, which should come at least 48 hours after the first workout in order to allow for sufficient recovery and strength gain.

Next, arrange for these students to work out only twice a week, on non-consecutive days, just like all the other kids. But instead of raising the bar and allowing them to jump, just keep the bar at the same height and expect them to perform one more repetition each week at the same level.

Kids Who are Obese Can't Do This

So for example, if you start week number one with 5 leg assisted pull-ups, in week number two they'll do 6, in week number three they'll do 7, etc. In this scenario, after one year, the student will be doing 57 leg assisted pull-ups (5 + 52). After year two, they'll be doing 109 leg assisted pull-ups. After year three, 158, and after year four they'll be doing 200 leg assisted pull-ups.

One Other Big Advantage

Actually in one very real sense, this is a better routine than the conventional routine because it requires so much leg/hips work. This in turn translates into muscle mass gain in the student's largest muscles. And muscle mass gains go hand in hand with an increased metabolism, anyone's most potent weapon against future fat gains.

Under these conditions the student who's predisposed to being unable to do conventional pull-ups will be so much more physically efficient than when he or she started that it will be literally impossible for them to be obese. And just like the kids who are doing conventional pull-ups, these kids will learn first hand how making a little bit of progress over a long amount of time, results in a mountain of success…physically and in every other way. They will have also immunized themselves against obesity for life as long as they maintain the little habit that you have ingrained into them at a young age.

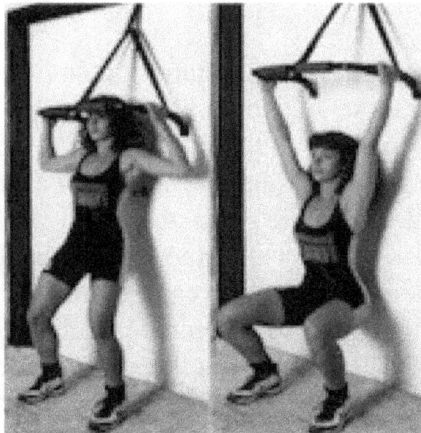

Conventional Pull-ups VS Leg Assisted Pull-ups

Here's a trick question for you. In which instance are you doing more physical work?

1. When you perform 10 conventional pull-ups *, or
2. When you perform 10 unconventional, leg assisted pull-ups in which you're allowed to keep your feet flat on the floor while your legs help you move your body up and down through the pull-up range of motion on the bar?

The answer of course is that you're doing precisely the SAME amount of physical work, moving the same exact weight through the same exact distance in both instances. Now the difficulty of doing that amount of work using only your arms in the conventional edition is much greater, because you're eliminating the leg assistance. And by adding your legs back into the equation the exercise becomes much easier. But in both cases though, the amount of physical work being performed is exactly the same.

With that said, why would anyone want to consider doing leg assisted pull-ups instead of conventional pull-ups? There are several good reasons. For starters the highest percentage of people these days are unable to do any conventional pull-ups, so the leg assisted variety gives these folks a viable point where they can begin and foundation upon which they can build.

But even if you're fully capable of performing conventional pull-ups you may still want to consider using the leg assisted variety simply because you can do so much more physical work when your les are part of your recipe. In my own case for example, I can do 8 or 10 conventional pull-ups in one set before I'm maxed out and I hit the fatigue wall. Then I have to rest for a minute or two before I do another set, etc.

But when I add in leg assistance I can perform 150 repetitions without stopping, at a pace of one rep per second. In other words I can do 5 to 15 times more physical work in the same amount of time or less, and that's a very interesting trade off in my book.

Secondly, with conventional pull-ups I get lots of great upper body pulling work and ZERO hips and legs work. But by adding legs to the mix, I not only get lots of great upper body pulling work, but I also get a ton of leg and hip work at the same time. In other words with leg assisted pull-ups I get lots more bang for the time and effort I invest.

One additional thought is that the intensity of 150 leg assisted pull-ups at a pace of one per second is so great that I also get a challenging cardio workout. In fact I dare anyone to do 150 leg assisted pull-ups at one rep per second without being pretty exhausted when they're done. It's much more challenging than it sounds. And if you add leg assisted dips you'll cover upper body pushing work in your routine as well. What a lethal and functional combination these two exercises are in my estimation.

(*) Dips can be substituted for pull-ups at any point in this chapter and it still works.

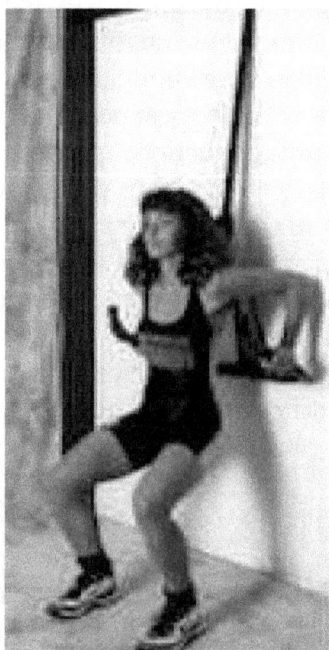

OPYOW With a Jump Rope

I have a friend named Dan Green who's in the fitness business. And as a member of the fitness community he kind of expects himself to maintain a certain level of physical fitness so that he's walking the walk as well as talking the talk.

But when we last met, I found that Dan was a little disappointed in himself in terms of the fitness level that he expects of himself, so he'd started a rope jumping program to counteract the problem. When he told me I congratulated him because I believe *when it's approached correctly*, jumping rope is a great way to improve fitness.

Keeping the Motivational Flame Burning Brightly

So what do I mean by, "When it's approached correctly?" Well, I'd wager that simply jumping rope several times a week will probably fall short of producing the results Dan's aiming for. Now don't get me wrong, doing something certainly beats doing nothing, and IF he keeps it up IT WILL YIELD RESULTS.

But the inevitable challenge is keeping it up because without regularity and longevity, no workout routine will get you to where you want to go. The big trick is to STAY MOTIVATED and to avoid having this year's good intentions being tossed into last year's pile of New Year's resolutions…foiled again.

The real question becomes how do you ignite that motivational flame and keep it burning week after week, month after month, and year after year? Interestingly enough it's really not all that hard… when you approach it correctly. Check it out.

Week After Week, Month After Month

Here's how you'd approach the problem in an Operation Pull Your Own Weight context. Start your program with a goal of producing documented progress week after week, month after month, all year long. In other words, you want to be able to honestly say to yourself (and anyone who's interested) that you really are a little better (i.e. physiologically younger, stronger, leaner) this week than you were last week, and a little better this month than last month, and lots better this year than you were last year.

For Example

For example, let's say that Dan starts out in week # 1 by rope jumping for five minutes, at a pace of 80 reps per minute. Then in each subsequent week let's say that he increases the pace by 5 reps per minute. So in week 2 he's up to 85 reps, in week 3 he's up to 90 reps, etc. Under these circumstances Dan expects to improve regularly for nine consecutive weeks before he hits 120 reps per minute (2 reps per second) which is a pretty decent pace for anyone who's not a professional boxer. Not only that but 120 reps per minute may be about all Dan can squeeze into 5 minutes worth of rope jumping.

A Tangible Return on Investment

Notice the motivating factor, the tangible return on Dan's investment of time and effort is his regularly documented performance improvement. Dan also knows that every weekly performance improvement directly reflects an improvement in his physical efficiency, body composition, and a reduced percentage of body fat.

In the words of an old track coach of mine, "Champ, you can't get faster and fatter at the same time. When you get faster your physical efficiency automatically improves." The old coach's observation is equally true for a 100 yard dash, a mile run, or five minutes worth of jump roping. Performance improvement reflects all kinds of good things for the performer.

So regardless of what the market is doing these days, if Dan's investment of time and effort is paying off handsomely, and he keeps coming back week after week, month after month with his motivational sails billowing and he's collecting his fitness dividends along with the compound interest that naturally accrues, it'll be a winner.

The Infinite Benefits of Relentless Persistence

Now let's broaden the lens a little and speculate on what happens if Dan carries this simple strategy forward for several years, improving week after week, month after month, and year after year. I don't know about you but my bet is that if Dan does anything close he'll end up with a black belt in rope jumping when he's done.

He'll also be lean and mean in a way that will turn most 25 year olds green (no pun intended) with envy. And he will have turned his physiological clock back week after week, month after month, and year after year. Now that's a pretty good return on your investment of time and effort, and a roadmap to transforming your original motivations and aspirations into what I like to call RELENTLESS PERSISTENCE.

And anyone who relentlessly persists at anything is inevitably destined to win ...no exceptions to the rule. And that's how you combine an Operation Pull Your Own Weight strategy with a jump rope and produce one big time winner.

STRONG
AT EVERYTHING
WEAK at
NOTHING

The Motivational Psychology of

Operation Pull Your Own Weight

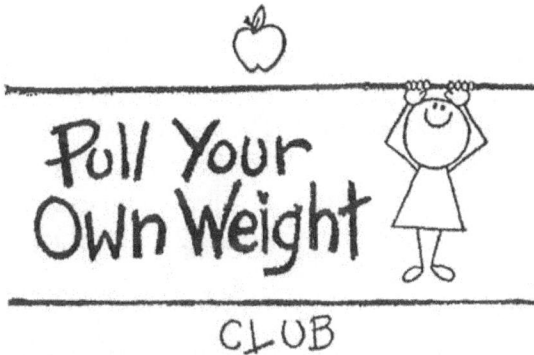

Motivating Kids To Take Action Against Obesity Today!

Multifaceted, complicated, and confusing are the kind of terms most experts currently use to describe the 21st Century childhood obesity dilemma. Arguably there are genetic, environmental, economic, sociological, and psychological factors that play a role in an issue the Attorney General of the United States has recently called "an epidemic, a pandemic, and a terrorist threat from within."

A Two Factor Dilemma...

On the other hand, when reality bashes in the door, all these complications can easily be boiled down to TWO FACTORS that we all understand. They are exercise and nutritional habits. In other words, there's not one American child who can't beat obesity by sufficiently raising their physical activity level and eating less/better.

Boiled Down to One Basic Challenge...

Childhood obesity prevention then can be boiled down to ONE basic challenge. Namely, how can we MOTIVATE kids exercise more and eat less/better? The fact is, even if their genes, environment, economics, social network or their psychological state make it harder for some children, any child who exercises enough and eats right will successfully avoid the 21st Century obesity trap.

And One Answer

That being the case, what motivates kids? The answer is, success always breeds success, and kids are no exception to this rule. Like an investor who experiences regular returns on his financial investment, kids who experience documented returns (in the form of regular progress) on their investments of time and effort, are MOTIVATED to continue investing as long as it continues to pay off. Consistently high levels of motivation translate into persistence. And relentless persistence is the key to success in anything, including childhood obesity prevention.

Let's Focus on One Example

Pull-ups for example, are very challenging for most kids today and they're impossible for kids who carry much excess weight because of the increased workload. But, if a bar is lowered to the point where the kid's feet are flat on the floor, there are very few kids who are unable to jump and pull themselves (their chins) up to the bar. This utterly simple technique is known as leg assisted pull-ups.

Inching Your Way Up

More specifically the strategy is to lower the bar to a level where a participant can EASILY do 8 leg assisted pull-ups, and allow them do a set of 8 reps. Working two days a week, say Mondays and Thursdays, the child comes back on day two (Thursday) and you allow them to do 9 leg assisted pull-ups. (1) In workout number three you allow them to do 10, in workout number four they do 11, in workout number five they do 12, and in workout number six THE BAR IS RASIED ONE INCH and the entire 8 to 12 routine is repeated all over, again and again until the child has run out of leg assistance and has mastered the ability to do conventional pull-ups.

Small Increments of Change

What I'd like to point out in this example is the extremely SMALL INCREMENTS OF CHANGE, that underwrite the extremely REGULAR EXPERIENCE OF PROGRESS, that translates into consistently HIGH LEVELS OF MOTIVATION, that eventually leads to RELENTLESS PERSISTENCE and eventual success at anything, including the ability to do pull-ups.

Success Magnified

The value of this experience in success can be magnified even further by conducting the activity in a social setting with other kids participating too. Then as kids make predictable progress workout after workout, week after week, month after month, their success is recognized and celebrated immediately with high fives from fellow participants and teachers who are supervising. It doesn't take long for kids to realize that successfully tackling a difficult task in public is FUN and they soon begin to look forward to their next opportunity to get stronger on the pull-up bar.

Motivation Embedded Into the Genetic Fabric

And as any gym teacher will attest, once any child has mastered pull-ups, they're naturally IMMUNIZED AGAINST OBESITY FOR LIFE as long as they maintain the ability, because people who can do pull-ups are NEVER OBESE.

But in the process, it's all about three things, MOTIVATION, MOTIVATION, and MOTIVATION. And the key to that vault is small, but regular increments of success, day after day, week after week, that over time, accumulate like compound interest in a bank and embeds the mantra "Oh Yes I Can" deep into the genetic fabric of any kid who's exposed to this life altering experience. May they all be exposed to this kind life altering experience at an early age.

(1) To be completely clear. The kids are ALLOWED ONLY 2 workouts per week. They're ALLOWED to do ONLY the number of pull-ups that are expected during that particular workout. Done this way you can INSURE that your kids experience progress (winning) every time they touch the bar for weeks and weeks in front of their friends and teacher. Under these conditions it doesn't take long before your kids are BEGGING FOR THE OPPORTUNTIY to do more pull-ups. WARNING, avoid giving in if you really want to keep those motivational flames burning brightly for a long, long time.

The Most Important Lesson a Kid Can Ever Learn is Best Taught Physically

I contend that one of the most important lessons any kid can ever learn is what I like to call the "Oh yes I can lesson." Whether they're male or female, black, white, yellow, Christian, Muslim, Jew, Asian, European, African, tall, short, rich, poor, or middle class, if kids develop their natural born ability to believe in themselves and to relentlessly persist, odds are they'll learn to succeed, even in the face of life's most difficult challenges, despite a system that's specifically designed to relentlessly mass produce infinite waves of mediocrity, homogeneity, predictability, conventionality, and submission to the status quo.

Show 'Em How

Now you may recognize this as the age old American adage that says "You can grow up to be President if you're willing to stick with it." But if this lesson is not delivered through practical, hands-on experiences (getting down in the mud and wrestling with the beast), it quickly becomes meaningless, adult doubletalk that goes in one ear and out the other for most kids. In other words, talk is cheap. The trick is to show them how to walk the walk if you really expect them to believe in themselves and to live their lives accordingly.

Show 'Em Early

Timing is also an extremely important consideration for the "Oh yes I can" lesson. In fact you have to get to them before they start school, because conventional school systems are so incredibly efficient at teaching kids the "Oh no you can't" lesson.

You see, school is specifically designed to pit kids against kids, expecting them to compete against one another for gold stars, teacher's praise, positions in the top reading or math group, who's the prettiest, who's the most athletic, who's the most popular, etc. By the time they're finished with first or second grade, most kids will have been thoroughly indoctrinated into the hierarchical mentality that sees the world in terms of a few winners at the top, the bulk of us (the masses) wrestling around in the middle, and a few stragglers (the kids term these days is "losers") bringing up the rear.

73

Immunizing 'Em Against the Bell Curve

In educational circles it's called the bell curve, and whether it's anywhere near true, most educators are paid to believe it, and to conduct their classes accordingly. If not immunized against this problem before they enter school, kids easily fall prey to the bell curve mentality, and they become passive victims of the machine that's built to convince most kids that they're average or worse, and there's very little they can do about it.

Conventional educators are of little help because most of them have lived with the bell curve for so long that it's second nature. And once the labels are systematically imbedded it's very difficult for kids to break out of the conventional box and to recognize that the system itself is stacked against them, fatally flawed, if not fraudulent.

However, if you teach kids to think for themselves, to see the world through their own eyes, and to relentlessly persist despite the system, many kids will survive, and their odds of living meaningful lives (real winning) are enhanced a thousand fold. They'll effectively be immunized against the system instead of indoctrinated by it. But remember, one of the biggest keys is to teach kids the "Oh yes I can" lesson before sending them off to school.

At the Physical Level

The third issue then is how to teach them what you want to teach them. My suggestion is that most young kids are far more physically oriented than they are mentally or spiritually oriented. And it's one thing to tell kids to persist and win, and an entirely different matter to physically show them how to persist and win. This is true whether they're going to be athletes or first cello in the county orchestra. The name of the game in the early years is PHYSICAL!

How About an Example

Ok, how about an example of what I'm talking about here. I suggest that you choose a body weight exercise that's generally associated with being strong. You see all kids want to be strong at everything and weak at nothing. It's in their genes. Have you ever met a kid who wants to be weak at anything? I know I haven't. Once you've chosen the strength oriented body weight exercise, then you simply help your kids learn to master it.

For example, everyone that I know associates pull-ups with strength, yet most kids today can't do pull-ups. However, if you start them young, before they've had a chance to super-size themselves, most kids can learn to perform pull-ups in a very predictable amount of time if they get the right advice and have access to the right equipment.

So consider the following scenario...
Your son, daughter, or student
- is going to set a difficult to achieve goal (to be able to perform pull-ups)
- is going to be given the right goal achieving information
- is going to be given access to the right goal achieving equipment
- they'll make a little progress every time they workout
- they'll be congratulated by peers and adults every time they progress (a great motivator!)
- they'll learn to look forward to the opportunity to grab hold of the bar and grow stronger
- within a few months they'll be able to do pull-ups (they'll reach their goal)
- they'll be immunized against obesity, because kids who can do pull-ups are never obese
- the more pull-ups they can do, the leaner they'll be. (Ma Nature designed us that way)
- they will be physically strong in a way that will impress friends and relatives
- but most importantly they will have learned all the above, first hand, at the physical level
- in other words, they'll have a first hand, physical experience in learning to control (take responsibility for) their own body (the physical self)

Expanding the Oh Yes I Can Lesson
Once this experience has been well chewed, digested, and understood at the physical level it will naturally expand to include everything else in a child's life from the three R's, to their social (a

positive self image is critical) and spiritual possibilities. With patience and relentless persistence, most children can reach almost any goal they set for themselves despite the system that's inadvertently working against them.

In simplest terms, if you don't think you can, you won't try. And if you refuse to try, failure becomes a predictable certainty. On the other hand, thinking you can always precedes genuine effort. Once under way, constant progress fans the motivational flames and keeps them burning brightly. And motivation is the fuel that feeds relentless persistence, the key to success.

Soaking it in Yourself

If you physically immunize your kids with the "Oh yes I can" lesson, on the physical level before you send them to school, you'll do them the biggest favor possible. You'll teach them the most important lesson they'll ever learn...to persist, persist, and persist again.

In the words of the late British Prime Minister Winston Churchill, "Never, never, never, never, give up!" In the words of former Olympic mile champion and world record holder Herb Elliot, "You've got to be arrogant enough to think you can, yet humble enough to pay the price."

There's really no substitute for relentless persistence. And teaching this lesson to kids is one of the surest ways to relearn it yourself.

Reagan, Obama, and the "Oh Yes I Can" Lesson

On the adult level, former President Ronald Reagan always maintained that his greatest achievement was to make the American people feel better about themselves in the wake of some pretty tough times. Ironically enough we currently have another guy named Barack Obama who's actively preaching the Oh yes we can lesson to Americans who are again wrestling with some pretty challenging times.

And just like their kids, American citizens who are convinced that they're helpless in the face of big money and big government, refuse to invest their limited time and effort into producing change. In other words they refuse to try. And those who refuse to try are the status quo's staunchest proponents. And they're easy to control, a dictator's dream.

The Best Time to Start is in Kindergarten

Democracy is completely dependent on citizens who believe that they must govern themselves and control of their own lives as opposed to being dictated to by autocratic bureaucrats. In this context, the "Oh yes I can" lesson lies at the very heart of American Democracy. And the best time to start learning it is in kindergarten.

But What Happens When the Going Finally Gets Tough?

A colleague recently wrote in and said, "I understand why you start each participant out at a level where they're guaranteed to succeed. I also understand why you use very small increments of progress/change, and restrict the amount of progress each participant is allowed to make in any one workout. And I understand why you want the leg assisted pull-ups to be done in front of the kid's peers and teachers."

"By doing these things you guarantee that all participants will experience a little success every time they workout for many workouts, and many weeks before things get very challenging. You're building in positive expectations, patterns of success experienced in public, storerooms of confidence producing psychological capital, and then you allow the resulting high fives from peers to motivate, inspire, and to help kids learn to look forward to their next opportunity to get on the bar and to get stronger."

But What Happens When the Going Gets Tough?

"What I fail to understand is what happens when the easy phase wears off and the whole thing becomes challenging. I mean learning to do pull-ups is tough for most kids these days. So I want to know what happens when the going gets tough?"

Excellent Question

First let me thank to my colleague for a great question. Now then, I confess, he's correct when he says that the easy phase eventually wears off and the whole thing inevitably becomes challenging for most kids. *I also understand that as a society, we've become too used to seeing kids giving up when the going gets tough, and refusing to try for fear of humiliating themselves in public.* Humiliation after all is un-cool, and all kids want to be cool and accepted by their peers. For most it's their highest priority.

But in four years of working with OPYOW I don't ever recall seeing even one child become discouraged and/or refusing to try. And the reasons for that certainly begin with the fact that we intentionally build public success into the experience. More specifically if the stage is set correctly each child will experience success (grow a little bit stronger) for many consecutive workouts, many consecutive weeks, and often for several months before things get real challenging.

Psychological Capital in the Experiential Bank

But eventually the going gets tough. It's inevitable. And when that happens each child should have weeks and weeks of public success under their belt. By this time the child should have a real good feel for what they're doing, and with an abundance of positive psychological capital stored up in their experiential banks (1) they can grab hold of the bar expecting to succeed just like they've done workout after workout, for weeks and weeks now.

Not only that, but the entire peanut gallery is expecting them to succeed because that's precisely what has happened every time they've touched the bar for a dozen weeks or more. Why should this time be any different?

The Peanut Gallery is Cheering Everyone On

The peanut gallery has also grown used to congratulating each participant when they're done, and they expect to do it again this time. That means they cheer and urge their peers to *keep on keeping on, especially when the going gets tough.* And when your friends are cheering you on it's really hard to give up, or to quit until you get your chin up to the bar just like everyone expects you to do.

The Psychological Chemistry is Suddenly Reversed

As a matter of fact, under these conditions, with everybody cheering you on, and expecting you to succeed, it's humiliating and it's un-cool to quit without giving it at least 1,000%. So you don't quit. You give it 1,000%. And when you do the odds of success are increased by approximately the same percentage.

Let me repeat this one more time so you don't miss it. Under these circumstances the psychological chemistry of pull-ups is suddenly reversed. *It's gone from REFUSING TO TRY for fear of being humiliated in front of your friends, to REFUSING TO GIVE UP for fear of being humiliated in front of your friends.* Now how cool is that?

79

An Increased Challenge Hardens the Resolve

As a matter of fact, in my experiences with OPYOW, when the stage is set right, an increased challenge produces an increase in the child's resolve to succeed. In other words when you're used to succeeding in public, and all your friends are expecting you to succeed in public, odds are that you're going dig down deep enough to find a way to continue succeeding in public.

It's cool to get stronger week after week, month after month. It's cool to be able to tackle a difficult task in front of your friends and succeed. And as the going gets tougher, the success becomes more fulfilling. Not only that but it's fun and you don't want to lose that fun, that cool, or that feeling of being a winner. And when you know the only thing standing between you and the goal line is a little more effort, it's not all that tough for most kids to dig down a little deeper and to come up with a little more.

It's All About Relentless Persistence

And in OPYOW, that's what happens when the going gets tough. We all come together. We all root for one another. And we all carry the ball across the goal line and celebrate each other's win because it's cool to be strong, it's cool to succeed, and it's really fun when we can all be cool, strong, and succeed together. When pull-ups finally evolve into a team sport, everyone wins. "Oh yes we do."

(1) With enough psychological capital stored up in their experiential banks, children can afford to risk hitting a bump in the road without fearing humiliation or embarrassment. As a kid once told me, "If I don't get it this time Coach, I'll get it next time. I promise."

Embarrassed When Talking to Kids About Obesity?

With childhood obesity growing exponentially, like a forest fire raging out of control, one big challenge for parents and teachers is to find ways to communicate with kids about the problem without offending or embarrassing them. After all, if you're unable to communicate, how can you resolve the problem? In light of that challenge, here are ten things to keep in mind when communicating with your kids on obesity.

1. Start young, before they have a chance to pick up too much excess weight. As a matter of fact, the younger you start, the better the odds become of avoiding childhood obesity, which almost inevitably turns into adult obesity.

2. Avoid negative terms like fat, obese, and chubby unless you want to offend the youngster's self perception, and all that goes along with it. That's a dead end street, with no redeeming qualities, and you should avoid it completely.

3. Instead, couch your conversations in terms of how to get stronger and avoid weakness. In many years of school teaching I met lots of kids who wanted to be bad, but I never met a kid (boy or girl) who wanted to be weak in anything (and that includes reading, writing, and arithmetic). Weakness in your kid's world is UNCOOL. However, BAD is just another way of saying strong, resilient, and uncompromising. So in place of good and bad, substitute strong and weak.

4. Choose an activity that pays for a child to get both stronger and lighter, and then teach them how to improve, in public, on a regular basis, over a period of time. Done correctly the child's public success, and the praise that follows, will show them that they can try new things in public (they can take a risk) without embarrassing themselves, feeling ostracized or alienated by failure. Done right, this activity will strengthen self-perception instead of undermine it.

81

5. This activity could take a variety of forms, but the simplest example is pull-ups. I suggest pull-ups for several reasons, starting with the fact that they're simple, everyone understands them, they require little space, and almost no money. Also most kids usually associate pull-ups with being strong.

6. And as any gym teacher will gladly confirm, kids who can do pull-ups are never obese. And kids who are obese can never do pull-ups. In other words, developing a kid's ability to do pull-ups, along with his/her desire to maintain it, immunizes them against obesity for a lifetime, naturally, without pills, shots, or special diets.

7. Using a height adjustable bar along with a technique called leg assisted pull-ups, where a child jumps and pulls at the same time, allows all kids to experience immediate and continued success. And by inching the bar higher and higher, they eventually run out of leg assistance and they're doing real live pull-ups.

8. Always treat pull-ups as an opportunity instead of an obligation. That is to say this activity should be something your kids get to do (like Disneyland) instead of something they have to do (like clean their room). It should be a reward not a job. Done right, you can use the opportunity to do pull-ups as the reward for cleaning their room. Until the room is clean Johnny, we'll do no pull-ups and you'll miss out on the opportunity to get stronger.

9. Lessons packed between the lines of this strategy include the fact that regular work, good eating habits, and getting sufficient rest (at night and in between workouts) MAKES A PARTICIPANT STRONG. On the other hand, the lack of regular work, poor eating and rest habits, along with counterproductive behaviors such as using tobacco, alcohol, and drugs MAKES A PARTICIPANT WEAK. And again, I've never met a child who wants to be weak in anything. Have you?

10. The other hands-on lesson that you can teach is personal responsibility. In other words if someone else does your homework on the pull-up bar, you make no gains. Nobody else can do the work for you...it's totally up to you.

P.S. What if you've failed to start 'em young before they've had a chance to pick up much excess weight? What if they're in junior high, high school or beyond, and they're already significantly overweight and deathly scared of anything that smells like a pull-up bar? What then?

The Golden Rule of Pull-ups

My suggestion is that the golden rule of pull-ups is equally true for kids from three to ninety three. That is to say if you can do pull-ups you can't carry much excess weight, and if you carry much excess weight you can't do pull-ups.

Almost Anyone Can Become...

However, almost anyone at any age can use a height adjustable bar together with leg assisted pull-ups to generate immediate access/success. Furthermore, almost anyone can inch the bar higher and higher over time, combining regular workouts with improved eating and rest habits, and produce thin slices of improvement over weeks and months until they can physically pull their own weight.

Immunized Against Obesity

And when they reach their goal, they've immunized themselves against obesity for a lifetime without pills, shots, or special diets, as long as they never lose that hard won ability. It's about that simple.

No You Can't, Oh Yes I Can: Teaching Kids to Stand Up to a Challenge

If you know your kids well enough here's a little game you can play with them while you're putting them through their Operation Pull Your Own Weight paces. I call it the "No you can't, Oh yes I can game," and here's how it goes.

Just before a student grabs the bar and begins doing their pull-ups, the overseeing adult says to him/her, "Johnny, I don't know if you're going to be able to do all those pull-ups today." The pre-arranged response from Johnny is to look the adult straight in the eye and say, "Oh yes I can," before proceeding to do the expected number of pull-ups. When he's done, Johnnie gets an immediate high five from the teacher and his peers, along with the experience of having successfully stood up in the face of a challenge.

Habitual Response

Yes, everyone will know the whole thing is completely staged, but if handled correctly, and repeated over weeks and months, this role playing experience becomes much more than just theatre. It's a practiced response that becomes a habit, a built in reaction that's almost ingrained into Johnny's regularly beefed up DNA giving him the psychological wherewithal and the confidence to confront a legitimate challenge (in this case pull-ups) and to expect success.

The Best Time

The best time to incorporate this game is in the second or third week of the program when you've established a starting point for all the participants, and when progress is relatively guaranteed for the next 8, 10, or 12 more weeks. In other words you want Johnnie to accept the challenge, and to succeed in public week after week, month after month. That's how it becomes a habit, and how the Oh yes I can attitude bleeds off into other parts of his life, such as his reading, writing, and his arithmetic.

Some Teachers Were Leery

Some teachers were a bit leery of this game, fearing the "Oh yes I can" response would turn into uncontrollable backtalk in the classroom. In their view, there's plenty of that in our nation's schools already without actively encouraging it.

My own experience is that when the kids know you're on their side, helping to make them a little stronger every week, every month, all year long, they naturally respect you and they'll keep a handle on their behavior in the classroom. It's the kids (and the teachers) who lack confidence who are threatened by a challenge and who lash out in the wrong ways. If teachers and kids are both confident, the result is mutual respect.

Wanna Put $50 Bucks On It?

I confess that on one occasion I had a little guy respond to my challenge by saying "You wanna put $50 bucks on that?" All the other kids got a good laugh, after which I said, "I'll put a nickel on it." The young lad went on to do his allotted number of pull-ups and happily took my nickel, along with my high five and congrats from the rest of his classmates. In the end, that kid turned out to be one of my best students, and he learned to say "Oh yes I can" to all kinds of challenges. Done it right, it works. Give it a try.

Motivating Kids by Engaging Them in Public Success

Picture this. On Monday Johnny (or Jenny, you choose) the Kindergartner (JTK) does 8 pull-ups at level one and gets a high five from the teacher along with his friends and classmates. On Thursday JTK does 9 pull-ups on the same level, followed by congrats and high fives all the way around.

The next Monday JTK does 10 pull-ups. Next Thursday he does 11. The following Monday he does 12, all followed by congrats and high fives every time. Next Thursday the bar is raised one inch, making his pull-ups a little harder so JTK does 8 pull-ups at this next level, with congratulatory high fives for moving up to the next level.

The Pattern Continues

Now consider that this pattern of success continues every workout for 8, 10, 12 consecutive weeks or more. My question for you is, *how do you think JTK feels about doing pull-ups?*

Realistically speaking, it's getting harder and harder with every workout, and every week. But Johnny continues to succeed despite the difficulty. In fact the increased difficulty combined with JTK's success might even make his focus, his interest, and his desire to perform even more intense. What do you think?

Learning to Expect Success?

Do you think that Johnny's learning to expect success on the pull-up bar? Do you suppose that his self confidence is growing with every passing week? Do you think that JTK may be learning to look forward to his next opportunity to get on the bar and to become stronger? Do you agree with me when I say that every kid I've ever met (I taught school for 17 years) wanted to be strong at everything and weak at nothing? Have you ever met a kid who wanted to be weak at anything? I sure haven't.

Immunized Against Obesity for Life

This motivational technique is why kids who participate in *Operation Pull Your Own Weight* learn to look forward to doing pull-ups. In the process they learn to be a little stronger this week than they were last, a little stronger this month than last, and a lot stronger this year than last. And by the way, kids who learn to do pull-ups have also learned to (naturally) immunize themselves against obesity because kids (people) who can do pull-ups can't be obese. Now let's take this scenario one step further.

What would happen if you applied this same motivational technique to JTK's reading, writing, and arithmetic? What would happen to his overall self confidence? What would happen to his ability to tackle a new challenge while expecting to succeed? What would happen when he finally experiences a bump in the road and needs to dig in to overcome it? Would he be more likely to persist and work his way through it?

Reading, Writing, and Arithmetic?
There's an old adage that says "Success breeds success." In other words, success builds on itself and kind of snowballs in all kinds of different directions.

Failure, interestingly enough, does precisely the same thing. What happens if Johnny learns that there's no return on his investment of time and effort in front of his friends? Worse yet, what if he learns that there's a negative return on his investment (i.e. failure and humiliation in front of his friends)?

Which of these experiences do you think that most kids are having in school these days? Maybe they could learn something from JTK and Operation Pull Your Own Weight. What do you think?

Using What All Kids Want… to Motivate Them to Eat Right, Exercise More, and to Naturally Immunize Themselves Against Obesity for Life!

Let's start off by asking, then answering the question "What do all kids want?" Now that's a pretty broad question I admit, but for our purposes the answer is, <u>all kids want to be strong at everything and weak at nothing</u>. Let me add, in 17 years of teaching physical education and coaching not once did I ever meet a kid who wanted to be weak at anything. Have you? Not only that, given the option, they'll all choose to be strong at everything, no exceptions.

This brings up another thing that all kids want. <u>They all want to avoid obesity</u>. In all my years of teaching I never met even one kid who actually wanted to be obese. I knew plenty of kids who suffered dramatically from being fat, but they didn't really know how to eliminate fat from their lives so they just suffered. In any case, all kids want to avoid obesity…bank on it.

Pull-ups and Strength

Let me ask another question. What do you associate with the ability to do pull-ups? If you said "strength," congratulate yourself because you're in the majority. People who can physically pull their own weight on a pull-up bar are inevitably considered physically strong. In fact President Obama recently accepted a pull-up challenge from a couple of his aids and proceeded to out-muscle them on the pull-up bar. <u>Pull-ups and strength go together</u> like oceans and waves, mountains and heights, catfish and whiskers. You can't have one without the other.

Pull-ups and Lightness

The other thing that pull-ups are always associated with is "lightness." Look at Obama. I mean have you ever seen even one obese person who can do a single pull-up? In my seventeen years of teaching and coaching I can honestly say that <u>kids who could do at</u>

88

least one pull-up were NEVER OBESE. And kids who were obese could never do a pull-up.

We Know Three Things

OK, so far we know the following. All kids want to be strong at everything and weak at nothing. All kids want to avoid obesity and would do so if they really knew how to get that job done. And we know that pull-ups are always associated with being strong and being light because kids who can do them are always physically strong, light, and they're never obese.

Cool VS Uncool

But there's one more piece to our motivational puzzle that needs exploring before we pull it all together, which is the fact that all kids want to be cool and to be accepted by their peers. So let's point out right now that being strong has always been cool, and being weak has always been uncool for all kids, regardless of generation, age, gender, race, religion, economics, ethnicity, etc.

And one way to prove your strength and your cool is to be able to tackle a difficult task in front of your friends and to succeed week after week, month after month, all year long. Success breeds success, as well as confidence, self worth, independence, etc. Now we're getting down to the motivational nitty gritty for all kids from sea to shining sea and around the world.

Introduce Kindergartners to…

Consider the following scenario. Introduce all kindergartners to a height adjustable pull-up bar together with a technique called leg assisted pull-ups (LAP's) where kids are allowed to jump and pull simultaneously in order to succeed at doing pull-ups. Lower the bar enough and all kindergartners will find a successful starting point for leg assisted pull-ups. In fact the starting point for each student should be a level where they can EASILY do 8 LAP's.

How Easy?

How easy you ask? It should be so easy that each participant WILL KNOW that they'll be able to do ONE MORE LAP in each of the next 5 workouts. That is to say in workout # 2 each student will be allowed to do nine reps (NO MORE), in workout # 3 ten, in workout # 4 eleven, and in workout # 5 twelve.

In workout # 6 the bar will be RAISED ONE INCH and the entire 8 to 12 scenario is repeated all over again for 5 more workouts, and 5 more workouts, and 5 more workouts until the participant has finally run out of leg assistance and has learned to do conventional pull-ups on their own, and feels a great sense of accomplishment over their achievement.

Small Increments of Change/Progress

The key thing to notice here is that the increments of change/progress are very small which puts kids in a position where they succeed workout after workout, week after week for 8, 10, or even 12 straight weeks or more. In so doing these kids develop patterns of success in which they learn to expect to succeed instead of expecting to fail. And when you expect to succeed your odds of trying hard enough to succeed increase exponentially. In the process the kids develop what I call a sense of Relentless Persistence which is the key to succeeding in anything from pull-ups to rocket science.

Less Than an Hour Per Week to Immunize 30 Kids

Workouts by the way take less than a minute per child including height adjusting the bar. This means that 30 kids can learn to succeed in front of their friends in less than an hour per week (2 workouts/week on non-consecutive days) and by year's end 90% of your kindergartners will have learned to do pull-ups and immunized themselves against obesity for life, and the other 10% will be well on their way to winning the battle.

Taking Full Advantage of What Kids Want to Help Them Win!

Repeat this scenario for five consecutive years and you will have eliminated childhood obesity in your school by taking full advantage of things that all kids naturally want, including:

- to be strong at everything and weak at nothing
- to avoid obesity and all the problems that accompany it
- and to grow strong and cool by tackling a challenging task in front of their friends, succeeding week after week, month after month, all year long, while celebrating each success with high fives and congratulations. How cool is that?

90

Selling "Cool" and Winning the Childhood Obesity War

In order to beat the childhood obesity epidemic in this country it would help if we introduced kids to an action plan that they would enthusiastically buy into. In other words, if kids are uninspired and they fail to buy into it, all the time, effort, energy, and resources we spend will be meaningless and inconsequential, not to mention a total waste of time and money.

The bottom line question in my mind is, are we insightful enough to come up with a program that kids will perceive as "COOL" so they'll be motivated enough to take action, so that we can finally turn the tide on childhood obesity? Here are a few thoughts on that question.

Bad vs. Strong and Weak

As an ex-teacher and coach I've met a lot of kids who take some pride in being bad. In fact today being bad is often considered the same as being cool. But in seventeen years of teaching and coaching I never met even one kid who took any pride in being weak at anything. In other words, every kid I ever met has wanted to be strong at everything and weak at nothing. How about you?

Here's What Being Bad Means

Lets' translate all this in a little different way. Saying "I'm bad" is a modern way for kids to say "I'm strong. I don't cave into teachers. I don't cave into parents. I don't cave into authority, the status quo. I stand my ground. I don't take crap from anyone, so don't mess with me." In this sense, being bad is cool, which makes it acceptable.

Strong is Always Cool

Historically speaking, being strong has always been cool, and being weak has always been uncool. In this light, and in their heart of hearts, every kid I've ever met longs to be strong and cool at everything, while weak and uncool at nothing. It's human nature. It's built into the genes.

So What...

What does this analysis have to do with beating childhood obesity you ask? I suggest that it points us towards at least one answer to the question we originally asked... "Are we smart enough to create a program that kids will perceive as cool so they'll be motivated enough to take action, and so we can finally turn the tide and defeat childhood obesity?"

It's As Simple as ABC

I have a good friend who I usually refer to as the old coach who contends that the cool solution to the 21st century childhood obesity crisis is as simple as A,B,C. Here's how his logic goes.

A. Kids who can physically pull their own weight (i.e. do pull ups) are never obese.

B. Start them young, allow them to use a height adjustable pull up bar and leg assisted pull ups, almost all kids can learn to do pull ups in a predictable amount of time and have a great time doing it.

C. If A and B are true, then it's also true that almost all kids can naturally immunize themselves against obesity for life by learning and maintaining the ability to do pull ups for a lifetime.

Graduates Who Pull Their Own Weight

In the coach's own words, "If we help kids learn to do pull ups starting in kindergarten, and help them maintain it through graduation, the childhood obesity epidemic would be ancient history in less than a decade. With that insight in hand, there are no longer any excuses for failing to turn the tide on childhood obesity.

It's simple. It's safe. It's cheap. It works for both boys and girls of any size, ethnicity, economic background, etc. And it's been proven to win enthusiastic approval from kids who all think it's extremely cool to be strong, and extremely uncool to be weak. What more can you possibly want?" I for one, always found it hard to argue with the old coach because he's usually right.

"Some Kids Want To Be Bad, But No Kids Want To Be Weak"

One of the important strategies of *Operation Pull Your Own Weight* is to **exchange the terms** good and bad, for the terms strong and weak in your child's vocabulary. Why you ask? In the seventeen years I spent teaching and coaching, I met plenty of kids who "wanted to be bad." But I never met one who "wanted to be weak."

Girls, Boys, All Ages…

That goes for girls as well as boys, regardless of age, race, ethnicity, religion, etc. Think about for a second, have you ever known anyone who actually wanted to be weak? Personally I've never known anyone, who ever knew anyone, who actually wanted to be weak. We all want to be strong. It's just how human beings are programmed. And for most kids, being able to perform pull-ups is a sure sign of physical strength.

What Does It Take?

But what does it take to develop strength on the pull-up bar? According to the OPYOW recipe it takes…
- regular work (twice per week),
- eating right,
- getting enough rest,
- and avoiding tobacco, alcohol and drugs.

In other words we taught kids that if they worked out on the pull-up bar a couple times each week, ate right, got sufficient rest, and avoided tobacco, alcohol, and drugs, they'd get stronger on the pull-up bar. We also taught kids that if they failed to work out regularly, if they ate poorly, failed to get enough rest, and messed with tobacco, alcohol, and drugs, they were shooting themselves in the foot, and asking to be weak.

No Way! That'll Make Me Weak!!!

In fact I had a kindergartner back in the Jefferson School days who, in front a class full of kids, looked up at me and said,

"Coach, my uncle Freddie wanted me to smoke a cigarette with him last night, but I told him, "No way. That'll make me weak." I immediately gave this youngster five, as did his teacher, and the rest of his classmates who all understood that messing with tobacco, alcohol, and drugs make you weak! And as we said previously, none of these kids wanted to be weak in anything.

Readin', Writin', and Rithmatic Too…..

Interestingly enough, those same kids who want to avoid weakness on the pull-up bar, also want to avoid weakness in all other aspects of their lives too, including their academics. And interestingly enough the habits that make you strong on the pull-up bar are the exactly the same habits that make you strong in every other aspect of life as well. If you work at reading (writin' or 'rithmatic) regularly, over a period of time, eat right, get plenty of rest, and avoid negative habits like tobacco, alcohol, and drugs, you'll eventually be strong in reading (writin' and 'rithmatic), taking it one step at a time.

In Conclusion…

In conclusion, done correctly, the lessons you teach on the pull-up bar carry over to all other aspects of a child's life because, as we've said a number of times now, some of them may want to be bad, but none of them ever want to be weak. If you make your case in these terms, your kids understand, they'll respond positively, and they will develop *not only physical strength, but an inner strength and confidence* (self esteem) in themselves and their ability to meet challenges, and to overcome obstacles. Is there a better lesson you can teach a child at a young age? Personally, I can't think of one.

An Open Letter to Kids Who Want to be Strong at Everything and Weak at Nothing

Dear Kids:

I'm a former teacher who spent 17 years teaching physical education and coaching various sports. I'm also a father who has two adult age kids - to me they're still kids just like you will always be to your Mom and Dad.

Bad, but Never Weak

One way or the other, in my sixty years, I've known lots of kids and I confess that I've never met even one who wants to be weak at anything. I've met lots of kids who will tell you they want to be bad, but never one who wants to be weak. Every kid I've ever known wants to be strong (independent and adult-like) at everything and weak (dependent and child-like) at nothing, and I presume you're no exception to the rule.

Strong Kids

In that light, I've also noticed that the kids who are really strong at lots of things are also confident, and they have no need of being pretentious about much of anything. They know who they are, and they're generally happy with that.

Weak Kids

On the other hand, kids who feel like they're weak in various ways, usually lack confidence and they often feel the need to pretend to be tough, defiant, and yes BAD. These kids feel threatened by other people, especially those who are different from them, and they hide behind all kinds of self erected walls and fences, including the way they dress, wear their hair, the music they listen to, and the way they interact with their parents, teachers, and peers.

The Antidote

These same kids still want to be strong at everything. But their feeling of weakness inhibits their ability to explore new

95

possibilities because they're scared of failing and being humiliated in front of their friends. It's much safer and easier to be able to claim, "I didn't try." At least there's a viable excuse for failure, and some degree of cool is maintained. The antidote of course is to start young and help these kids learn to become strong at all kinds of things. Under these conditions the walls and fences of pretension are never erected.

A Friend?

Now let me ask you a question. If you knew an adult - a teacher or a parent - who would help you learn to become a little bit stronger every day, every week, every month, all year long, would you have lots of respect for that person? Would you be inclined to listen to that person's advice, and follow it because you know it'll make you stronger? In the long run, could an adult like this even turn out to be your friend?

Every Day, Week, Month

Let's take this conversation in a little different direction. Do you know any kids who make a practice of growing a little stronger every day, every week, every month, all year long? If someone actually did that, starting at a young age, right on into adulthood, can you imagine just how strong that person would actually become? If you did that starting at a young age, can you imagine how strong you'd be? Can you imagine how confident you'd be? Can you imagine how unique, how interesting, and how cool you'd be?

What's Important to You?

I guess the important question now is, "What's really important to you?" Given the opportunity, in what ways would you like to become strong? Would you like to have a strong body that allows you to run fast, jump high, move quickly from side to side, climb ropes, mountains, etc? Would you like to have a strong mind with which you can think, calculate, understand, read, and write creatively and productively? Would you like to have a strong spirit that gallops to the top of the hill each morning, mane and tail flowing in the breeze, rearing up, silhouetted against the horizon in which your mind and body merge and express your admiration and appreciation to Mother Nature? God? Life?

Relentless Persistence, the Key of Keys

In order to experience life at this level, you must first recognize that you can become a little stronger every day, every week, every month, every year, for many years running. You must also recognize that you can progress regularly, if you take small bites, designed to continually reignite your motivation, resulting in a lifelong pattern of Relentless Persistence. Finally, you must recognize that through Relentless Persistence, almost any goal can be reached by almost anyone who wants to be strong at everything and weak at nothing.

Instant and Delayed Gratification Built Into the Same Childhood Obesity Package

Teaching kids to immunize themselves against obesity by teaching them to perform pull-ups (obese kids can't do pull-ups) with a height adjustable pull-up bar (HAPUB) and leg assisted pull-ups (LAPU's) provides instant and delayed gratification in the same package. Check out the strategy and the childhood obesity prevention technique in *Operation Pull Your Own Weight.*

Height Adjustable Pull-up Bars and Leg Assisted Pull-ups

Using a height adjustable pull-up bar allows students to start with their feet planted firmly on the ground in order to perform leg assisted pull-ups, where they're encouraged to jump and pull at the same time. The bar is placed low enough that participants can do at least eight leg assisted pull-ups in their first workout, succeeding right away in front of their peers, creating immediate gratification.

Learning to Love Pull-ups

In workout number two *they're allowed* to do nine, in workout number three they do ten, in workout number four they do eleven, and in workout number five they do twelve leg assisted pull-ups. When they can do twelve LAPU's, the bar is *raised one full inch*, and the entire eight to twelve repetition scenario is repeated all over again.

Done correctly most participants will improve just a little bit, every single time they workout for eight or ten weeks straight. In the process they lose their fear of the pull-up bar and actually learn to look forward to their opportunity to perform successfully, in public.

Instant Combined With Delayed Gratification

By using the height adjustable pull-up bar together with leg assisted pull-ups, students can literally "inch their way up towards the ultimate goal of doing real live, conventional pull-ups. The long-term goal of being able to do pull-ups often takes weeks, months, or even a year to complete. *This translates into delayed gratification.*

But on the way to reaching that ultimate goal, the regular, but thin slices of success provide the immediate gratification, fan the motivational flame, and teaches participants to "expect success" (confidence/self esteem) not failure. It also teaches them to persist, persist, and persist in order to achieve that ultimate goal that they've set for themselves.

It Works With the Three R's Too

Interestingly enough the "thin slices of success strategy," with its built in instant and delayed gratifications, works not only for pull-ups, but for reading, writing, and arithmetic too. Educators who successfully teach kids to understand their experience on the pull-up bar, can easily *translate that experience into the academic arena.* In the process they'll cultivate self confident and highly motivated kids who can handle delayed gratification and immunize themselves against obesity at the same time, as long as they maintain the ability to do pull-ups.

Check Out the Return on Investment, and Compound Interest of Physical Fitness

When you ask kids to exercise more and eat better/less in the name of obesity prevention, you're asking them to invest their time, energy, and self images into doing these things. And like any other investor, kids expect to see a return on their investment if they're going to continue investing.

Increasing the Odds of Investment

In other words, if they can see regular documented proof that their investment is paying off, week after week after week, the odds of them continuing to invest is increased significantly. If the frequency of that improvement drops to month after month after month, some of the wind will drop out of their motivational sails. But if they have to wait three months, six months, or a year before seeing tangible proof that their investment is yielding a profit, odds are you'll lose them completely.

So the key to keeping a strong wind in their motivational sails is regular, frequent, documented progress - a tangible return on their investment of time, energy, and self image. However, if you can produce that kind of frequent and positive feedback, another factor comes into play. This factor I like to call The Compound Interest of Fitness.

Interest Compounding on Itself

Because of its unique ability to transform a little money into a lot of money, Albert Einstein, (among others) called compound interest "The eighth wonder of the world." It does this by allowing interest to be charged on interest, (interest compounding on itself) which grows the original asset exponentially. In this light, I contend that physical fitness has the same compounding effect on people.... especially kids.

In the Physical World

In other words, show me a kindergartner who can run like the wind, jump like a rabbit, move quickly from side to side, climb a tree or a rope, and I'll show you a kindergartner who's brimming with self confidence. That confidence in turn spills over into their social relationships, their ability to try new things, including reading, writing, and arithmetic, and almost everything else in their young, impressionable lives. It's totally natural and in the genes.

On the other hand, show me a kindergartner who's unable to run, jump, move quickly, and climb trees and I'll show you a kindergartner who lacks the confidence of his naturally confident counterpart. And that lack of confidence also spills over into their social relationships, their ability to try new things, including reading, writing, and arithmetic, and almost everything else in their young, impressionable lives. That too is natural and in the genes.

And in the Lives of Our Kids

The moral of this story is that when young kids are exposed to experiences in which they get regular, and predictably positive returns on their investments of time, energy, and self image, they'll continue to invest (they'll relentlessly persist) week after week, month after month, and year after year. And if they relentlessly persist week after week, month after month, year after year they'll grow stronger and stronger at whatever it is they're investing in, whether it's their body, their social relationships, or their academic performance.

If we make sure that all kids are exposed to these kinds of regular, positive experiences we'll raise a generation of kids who will grow up to be strong, responsible, self reliant, and resilient human beings. As parents, educators, and citizens, how can we justify giving our kids anything less than a regular return on their investments, and helping those investments to earn boatloads of compound interest?

Just Like Your Kids, Rufus is a Natural Born Runner

My dog Rufus loves to run. He's a snow white, 27 lb. Jack Russell Terrier who's so full of energy that he's hard to appreciate without seeing him in action. He spends a good percentage of his life suspended in mid-air (some call it levitation?) in between vertical leaps (some call it Michael Jordan) that lifts him eyeball to eyeball with his humans…my wife and me. But given the opportunity, Rufus is so affectionate that he'll lick your face off. He also loves to chase squirrels and cars, which is why we keep him leashed when we go out to take care of official business.

Rufus Loves Running Free

But on good weather days (excluding winters here in Chicago) we take Rufus across the street in back of Butterfield Elementary School where there are several acres with no streets for him to dash into, and no cars for him to chase after. In that setting we unleash the Rufmeister and allow him to do what he loves to do…run freely. His coloring helps us spot him at a distance. He also comes when called, so safety is a non-issue.

Once off the leash Rufy runs at various speeds, stops and sniffs some tantalizing tidbits, and then he takes off running again. And once in a while a neighbor named Russ brings his Brittany Spaniel named Tigger out at the same time. The fun these two dogs have running, chasing, sniffing, tumbling all over each other is a sight to behold.

We Didn't Teach Rufus to Love Running…

Now let me make one quick observation. We didn't teach Rufus to love running and Russ didn't teach Tigger to love running either. Loving to run came naturally to both dogs. It's built into their genes, which is the case for all dogs so far as I know.

Sure, I've seen the occasional, overly domesticated dogs who are fat and waddle from place to place. But they're probably older, and have undoubtedly spent most of their days inside, lying around in front of the TV snoozing. However, if you start 'em young, and give 'em the opportunity to develop naturally, it's perfectly normal for dogs to love running and romping… <u>just like your kids love it</u>.

It's In the Genes, Just Like Your Kids…

Learning to run follows in sequence just after learning to walk. Once walking is mastered, dogs and kids automatically want to speed up, which is when running is first experienced. Think about this. Have you ever seen the look of sheer ecstasy on a child's face at the moment they realize they're walking…and then again when they realize they're running? And when other kids show up to play, the feeling of ecstasy is amplified while they run and romp just like Rufus and Tigger in back of the school.

I agree that kids must first be safe before you unleash them. But if that ecstasy they experience when first learning to walk, and run is carefully cultivated over weeks and months for the first several years of their life, you'll find that your kids will gradually increase their love of running. As a natural byproduct, they'll also burn plenty of calories, develop good muscles, hearts, and lungs, have lots of fun, and eliminate stress, all without you having to teach anything. Given the opportunity, they'll learn on their own.

The Big Mistake

In fact the big mistake is when we adults try and teach our kids to run. We pit them against one another creating winners and losers. Or we encourage them to run around and around some school yard marathon style, bore them to tears, and create more winners and losers. And worst of all is when the gym teacher, a.k.a. the local high school football coach, uses running as punishment. "Give me two laps you slacker." Sound familiar? A better way to undermine anyone's natural love of running is hard to imagine.

Sometimes the system can be incredibly good at taking something that's an opportunity (I get to run) and transforming it into an obligation (I have to run), while sucking out every ounce of joy and fun, and turning it into sheer drudgery. Is it any wonder that our kids are getting fatter by the second? The big question becomes *how do we correct our mistakes*?

Let Them Run, Don't Make Them Run

The first part of that correction is to *begin to see running* (or anything else you want a child to learn) as a privilege, as *something they get to do* instead of an obligation, *something they have to do*. The second part is to *relentlessly cultivate that natural desire* by giving your kids the opportunity to expand on their initial experience (i.e. to learn more) safely, and celebrate every little improvement they make.

Given that opportunity and related support, they'll naturally learn to be a little better this week than they were last, a little better this month than last, and a lot better this year than last. Given the opportunity, that's how kids grow naturally.

In other words, give them the opportunity to learn what you want them to learn (running in this case) and you'll have to teach them very little. They'll experiment and soak up their experiences like the natural born sponges that they are. So if you let them learn, and avoid forcing them to learn, you'll be amazed at how much your kids will pick up naturally, and how little you'll have to teach them.

Running Compliments Pull-ups

One more point I'd like to make. Running compliments Operation Pull Your Own Weight very nicely by burning calories and helping kids keep their weight under control. And of course the lighter they are, the more efficient they'll be on the pull-up bar. It all kind of hangs together naturally because Mother Nature kind of planned it that way.

My Motivation: An Ode to Teaching

I never feel so strong and confident as when I'm helping kids to find their own strength and confidence. That's my motivation with Operation Pull Your Own Weight.

In a very real sense it's selfish. I'm doing it because I feel so good about myself when I'm doing it. The vibes of appreciation I receive when those kids get stronger and stronger, week after week, and more and more confident in their own natural abilities to set a goal and achieve it in small but relentlessly persistent increments of progress is unique in my life. Under these circumstances, I suddenly feel like Superman, Batman, Spiderman, Indiana Jones, Wyatt Earp, Muhammad Ali, Tiger Woods, and Elvis all combined in the eyes of these kids. I am unique in their lives.

If I Got This Kind of Lift From...

If I got the same kind of lift from climbing some corporate ladder, from running for public office, or from anything else, I'd be climbing a corporate ladder, running for public office, or doing something else that gives me the same amount of return on my investment of time and effort. But to date, nothing else compares.

There's no thrill of victory like the one I experience when seeing a young boy or girl learning to say "Oh yes I can," in the face of a real challenge, tackling it with unreserved enthusiasm, giving it 110%, having learned, and knowing in their heart of hearts that if they relentlessly persist, they will inevitably cross that finish line.

In the words of the late Winston Churchill, "Never, never, never, never, never, give up!" Not quitting is one very important form of winning. It's not the size of the dog in the fight, but the size of the fight in the dog that counts.

The Moment They Catch Their First Glimpse...

And the moment a child catches their first glimpse of the potential sitting out there on their own personal horizon, as long as they get a little stronger every week, every month, every year, is the moment they start approaching life in a different way, with a different attitude, with an excitement and an enthusiasm that was never there before. Let's just say, "For most everything else there's Master Charge."

And by the way, when I say kids, I'm talking about kids from 3 to 93. The fact of the matter is, when you help someone become stronger and more confident, no matter how old they are, you will have created a relationship that's unique. There aren't that many people in anyone's life who produce that kind of experience. And if you're one of them you will stand out from the crowd. You will hold a unique position in the life of that person, whether they're an elementary school student, or a rock and roll star.

The Clock Keeps on Ticking

So in answer to all those folks who have wondered why the OPYOW clock keeps on ticking inside me, it's because doing it makes me feel so good about me. To repeat my original statement, I never feel so strong and confident as when I'm helping kids to find their own strength and confidence. So there, I've said it out loud. If that were not the case, I'd be unable to persist. The flame would flicker and die. But it has not and now you know why. It's all about me and how it makes me feel about myself.

The Appendix

Operation Pull Your Own Weight

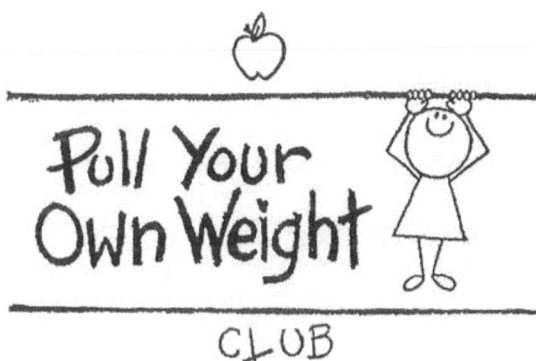

The PYOW Strong/Weak Test

1. All kids want to be…
   a. Strong and Independent
   b. Weak and Dependent

2. No kids want to be…
   a. Strong and Independent
   b. Weak and Dependent

3. Being strong and independent is about the same as…
   a. Being cool
   b. Being uncool

4. Being weak and dependent is about the same as…
   a. Being cool
   b. Being uncool

5. Some kids think it's cool to be…
   a. Bad
   b. Weak and dependent

6. But no kids think it's cool to be…
   a. Bad
   b. Weak and dependent

7. Learning to do pull-ups helps to make you…
   a. Strong, independent, and cool
   b. Weak, dependent, and uncool

8. When doing pull-ups it helps if you are…
   a. Heavy
   b. Light

9. The more pull-ups you can do…
   a. The stronger and lighter you must be
   b. The heavier and weaker you must be

10. If you want to learn to Pull Your Own Weight (to do pull-ups) it helps to…
    a. Practice regularly
    b. Eat better
    c. Do plenty of walking running to burn off calories
    d. Get enough sleep at night
    e. Avoid using tobacco, alcohol, and drugs
    f. All of the above
    g. None of the above

11. When learning to do pull-ups…
    a. It helps if someone else does the pull-ups for you
    b. You have to do the work yourself…nobody else can do it for you

12. As long as you maintain your ability to perform pull-ups…
    a. You'll never be obese, and you'll always be relatively strong
    b. You'll always be obese, and you'll never be strong

13. The habits that make you strong on the pull-up bar…
    a. Make you strong in all kinds of ways, including your school work
    b. Make you weak in all kinds of ways, including your school work

14. If you fail to make progress on the pull-up bar…
    a. It's the teacher's fault
    b. It's your parent's fault
    c. It's your friend's fault
    d. Take responsibility for yourself and failure will be a thing of the past

15. If you're too much overweight
    a. You will be unable to do even one pull-up
    b. You must be a girl

16. If you can do at least one pull-up…
    a. You can't be much overweight

b. You can't be a boy

17. If you can do lots of pull-ups…
    a. You have to be pretty strong and pretty light
    b. You have to be a girl

18. Using <u>tobacco</u> makes you…
    a. Weak and dependent
    b. Strong and independent

19. Using <u>alcohol</u> makes you…
    a. Strong and independent
    b. Weak and dependent

20. Using <u>drugs</u> makes you…
    a. Weak and dependent
    b. Strong and independent

21. <u>Eating poorly</u> makes you…
    a. Strong and independent
    b. Weak and dependent

22. <u>Allowing someone else to do your homework</u> makes you…
    a. Strong and independent
    b. Weak and dependent

23. <u>Getting too little sleep</u> at night makes you…
    a. Weak and dependent
    b. Strong and independent

24. The <u>simplest way</u> to make sure you're always strong, light, and cool is…
    a. Learn, and always maintain the ability to do pull-ups
    b. Wait until a big pharmaceutical company creates a magic pill
    c. Buy exercise equipment from a TV infomercial
    d. Learn, and always maintain the ability to do pull-ups
    e. A and D

The PYOW Strong/Weak Food Test

Here's a quick quiz you can give your kids to see it they can distinguish foods that make them strong and foods that make them weak. Alongside each food on the list have students write either the letter "S" for Strong food or the letter "W" for Weak food. Give it a try and see how your kids do.

1. Apples

2. Green beans

3. M and M's

4. French Fries

5. Strawberries

6. Milk

7. Pizza

8. Water

9. Frosted Flakes

10. Eggs

11. Snickers Bar

12. Salmon (fish)

13. Grape Jelly

14. Beef

15. Chocolate cake

16. Pancakes

17. Cheese

18. Peanut butter

19. Maple Syrup

20. Whoppers

21. Pickles

22. Ice Cream

23. Lettuce

24. Potatoes

25. Cabbage

26. Pineapple

27. Blueberries

28. Carrots

29. Cantaloupe

30. Water Mellon

31. Sugar

32. Butter

33. Oatmeal

34. Yogurt

35. Coca Cola

36. Peaches

37. Peach Pie

38. Chocolate chip cookies

39. Marshmallows

40. Hot Dogs

41. White Bread

42. Licorice

43. Peanuts

44. Pretzels

45. Capn' Crunch

46. Chicken breast

47. Pork

48. Hershey bars

49. Snow Cones

50. Mountain Dew

51. Pepsi Cola

52. Bananas

53. Oranges

54. Rice

55. Broccoli

56. Spinach

Don't be surprised when most of your kids get most of these questions right. Kids generally know the good foods from the bad foods, and if given the opportunity to choose good food on a regular basis, most kids will do so.

Strong Table, Weak Table: A Nutritional Experiment You Can Try With Your Kids

Here's a simple nutritional experiment you can try with your kids at home, or a teacher could do it in the classroom. Set up two tables. On one table place fruits, vegetables, and colorful photos of other food that's good for you like lean meat, fish, poultry, and dairy products. Then hang a sign on this table that reads "STRONG FOOD."

On the other table place candy, soda pop, sugary cereals, chips, and colorful photos of pizza, French fries, ice cream, and other things that are bad for you. On this table hang a sign that reads "WEAK FOOD."

Let Them Snack At Will

Then allow your kids to snack at their discretion from either table. My bet is that it won't take long before all the snacking is being done from table number one, and all the garbage food is being avoided like the plague. The reason I say that is, during my seventeen year teaching career, I met plenty of kids who took some pride in being bad. But I never met even one kid who took any pride in being WEAK at anything.

Automatically, Voluntarily

When kids really understand that eating the right foods makes you strong, and eating the wrong foods makes you weak, they start making the right choices automatically, voluntarily, without anyone lecturing them about anything. It'll happen all by itself as a matter of course, naturally. And that's exactly the way it should happen. To repeat myself one more time, there's not a kid in the universe who wants to be weak at anything. They all want to be strong at everything. Let's help them reach that goal.

Great Publicity With PYOW TV

Operation Pull Your Own Weight is all abut motivating kids to eat better/less, and exercise more. And as we've said on several previous occasions, small but regular increments of progress serve as the keys to keeping the motivational flame burning brightly over time, resulting in relentless persistence, which eventually leads to winning.

Media Motivation

But there's another important form of motivation that can be used to maximize the kid's motivational flame and to inform the public. Publicity handled right, transforms the local community into a chorus of supportive voices, and it gives your kids an extra boost when they see themselves or their friends on the pages of the local newspaper or being interviewed on the TV. It serves to reinforce the perception that learning to pull your own weight is an activity that's important, one to be valued.

The You Tube Advantage

But back in the 90's we didn't have access to the Internet, to websites, and we certainly didn't have anything even remotely similar to You Tube. With these thoughts in mind let me tell you what I suggest for a modern, simple, yet highly effective 21st century publicity strategy.

I suggest you take a video camera and film one entire session – a class going through their OPYOW paces – translate it into a You Tube presentation and post it on all your school's websites including the PTA and various booster clubs.

Monthly You Tube Installments

Do this once a month for each class that you're working with, and allow each participant to tell the camera how much progress they've made over the past month. Make sure and capture the camaraderie, the high fives from peers congratulating each other on their success. And if the teachers participate get that on camera too.

Let the Media Post It

Then tell the local media about your OPYOW You Tube postings and ask if they'd like to post them on their respective websites. They will take you up on it and it will plant a seed that will cause them to send reporters in droves out to cover your activities in the paper, the radio, and the local television stations(s).

Let Local Businesses Post It

If you want to take it a step further, let local businesses know about your OPYOW You Tube postings and ask if they'd like to post them on their websites as a sign of support. This will cause local businesses to be aware of your program and will increase the likelihood of their supporting you in other ways...i.e. T-shirts for your kids at the end of the school year?

Immunized Against Obesity for Life

By making the local community aware of what you and your kids are doing in the name of childhood obesity prevention you will benefit, your school will benefit from basking in the glow of positive publicity, and your kids will benefit by naturally immunizing themselves against obesity for life by simply maintaining the ability to do pull-ups throughout adulthood.

Everyone's Welcome to Join In

Finally, we welcome any OPYOW You Tube postings. We will soon be posting them on www.pullyourownweight.net and giving you, your school, and your kids national exposure. Who knows, maybe President Obama will call you one of these days in order to observe your kids pulling their own weight.

The Democratizing Effects of Immunizing Kids Against Obesity for Life, Starting in Kindergarten, (and Eliminating the Class Bully)

One of the most interesting and far reaching aspects of OPYOW is that kids who'd normally be left behind because they're genetically (or socially, psychologically, economically, etc.) predisposed to picking up excess weight will avoid being left behind because they'll immunize themselves against obesity for life by learning and maintaining the ability to do pull-ups. The confidence boost that results from this experience alone is beyond calculation. But there's more. Check it out.

Nothing Succeeds Like Success

When all kids learn at an early age that THEY CAN tackle a difficult task like learning to do pull-ups (Oh yes I can), in front of their peers, and when they succeed, week after week, month after month, every time they touch the bar, they learn to expect success instead of failure. Since nothing succeeds like success, those expectations spill over into the way they approach things like reading, writing, and arithmetic, so their academic performance benefits as well.

Embedded In a Kid's Psychological DNA

So, even those kids who are naturally athletic and can pull their own weight anyway learn to encourage everyone instead of just those at the top of the pecking order. It also influences how all the kids approach social relationships and it reduces the odds of there ever being a class bully (a kid dictator). They all learn patience, planning, persistence, and mutual respect, and those characteristics color the way they interact with the world around them forever.

Meanwhile, the gap between those kids who are naturally at the top of the pecking order and those who are at the bottom is significantly reduced, and the playing field is systematically leveled by RAISING STANDARDS for one segment, NOT LOWERING

THEM for another. And if all this begins at a young age when experience tends to become imbedded into kids' psychological DNA's, they'll carry over and last the rest of their lives.

Disruptive Behavior Will Diminish

With the playing field leveled and the pecking order gap systematically reduced, the negative experiences that cause many kids to feel frustrated, ashamed, angry, cynical, ostracized, embarrassed, humiliated, and alienated will be significantly reduced. And at this point the face saving, defensive behaviors that disrupt so many classrooms will diminish simultaneously.

As Performances Improve

And with disruptive behaviors minimized and student confidence levels enhanced, focus as well as performance levels will naturally improve and the democratizing chemistry resulting from OPYOW being introduced at an early age will make school, the community, and the world a more democratic place in which to live, work, and play.

Saluting the Flag of Democracy

Although OPYOW normally focuses in on childhood obesity prevention, that doesn't mean the ripple effects of solving one very big problem won't influence the lives of participants in an infinite number of other ways. And by making school, the community, and the world a better place, those natural athletes who are already predisposed to being strong, light, and well coordinated will also stand to benefit dramatically from the democratizing effects of OPYOW. And for those of us who salute the flag of democracy, that's a move in the right direction.

A Simple, Cost Effective Childhood Obesity Prevention Strategy For Any U.S. School District

Even though the childhood obesity epidemic has recently been described as leveling off, the problem is not subsiding, and we're light years away from eliminating it. While complicated and expensive solutions are being proposed by many authorities, one group of concerned exercise physiologists has recently outlined a simple 7 step solution that any school district in America can initiate, as long as they're action oriented, and they really want to take regular, documented bites out of childhood obesity in their own schools starting this fall.

Here's Their Simple 7 Step Solution....

1. Adopt a district wide goal of eliminating childhood obesity in one decade or less.

2. Conduct a district wide test to find out which of your students can perform conventional pull-ups. Since it's common knowledge that kids who can do conventional pull-ups can't be obese, you'll be starting off the school year off with documented evidence that a specific percentage of your students are not obese. This will serve as a baseline.

3. Reward all students who can perform conventional pull-ups with a special T-Shirt (sweatshirt, cap, etc.) and a Certificate of Immunization signifying that as long as they maintain their ability to do pull-ups, they'll be naturally immunized against obesity.

4. Encourage these students to increase their ability to do conventional pull-ups because the more pull-ups students can do, the greater their physical efficiency (leanness) will be.

5. Then, using a simple height adjustable pull-up bar and leg assisted pull-ups, begin to help all K-2 students learn to do conventional

119

pull-ups in a predictable amount of time, and to naturally immunize themselves against obesity in the process.

6. Each subsequent school year add one class level (i.e. in year 2 add 3rd grade, year 3 add 4th grade, etc) until all grade levels, K-12, are included.

7. Document and celebrate all your successes on your school's websites, and newsletters and keep the local media updated as you make regular, documented progress towards eliminating childhood obesity in your school district every day of the week.

If you like ideas that are simple, affordable, and proven, wait no longer. Take action today!

And a Potential State Budget

As indicated above, this simple cost effective obesity prevention strategy is one that any school district in the U.S. can initiate starting this fall if they're action oriented self starters. But if self starting, action oriented school districts are hard to find, some states may decide that it's time to pro-actively step in and prime the pump, and the following represents a State Budget that would start the ball rolling.

1. One State Director, $100,000 (total $100,000)

2. Ten Regional/County Directors at $50,000 each (total $500,000)

3. Ten $10,000 stipends to 10 physical educators per Region (10 stipends times 10 regions times $10,000 = $1,000,000)

4. Equipment and Publicity $400,000 (total $400,000)

5. Total State Budget (personnel, equipment, and publicity) $2,000,000

Project Goals

1. To document 20,000 students per state who are naturally immunized against obesity for life in year 1

2. To document 2,000 students per region who are naturally immunized against obesity for life in year 1.

3. Document 200 students per stipend holder who are naturally immunized against obesity for life in year 1.

4. Keep the average cost of naturally immunizing students against obesity for life to under $100 per student

5. Duplicate this project each year for one full decade at which point childhood obesity will be eliminated in this state.

6. A national budget (50 states) of $100,000,000 per year will produce/document at least 1,000,000 kids who are naturally immunized against obesity each year.

7. A decade long, national budget of $1,000,000,000 (one billion dollars over 10 years) eliminates childhood obesity in America and proves to be a veritable bargain when compared to the cost of failing to win that critical and costly war.

A Salute to Relentless Persistence:
Oh Yes We Can

His Dad was black and his Mom was white, and they divorced when he was still a baby so he grew up a mixed race child in a single parent home. Such a combination has turned many a child bitter, cynical, and angry enough at the world to stop trying, throw in the towel, and escape into booze, drugs, and violence.

Stronger Week After Week

But with constant encouragement from his Mom and his grandparents who were from Kansas, he avoided the bitterness, the cynicism, and the anger which has ensnared so many, and he replaced them with inner strength, optimism, and Oh Yes I Can. He was a relentless competitor who competed mostly with himself. His goal was always to be a little stronger this week than he was last week, a little stronger this month than last month, and a lot stronger this year than last year. He was absolutely relentless in his persistence, and week after week, month after month, year after year he grew stronger physically, mentally, and spiritually.

Colleges and Universities Welcomed Him

At the end of his high school years he discovered that his relentless persistence had opened up all kinds of educational opportunity and he had a plethora of good colleges and universities who were welcoming him into their midst. He chose to attend Columbia University in his undergraduate experience and Harvard for graduate school, all the while continuing to grow stronger and stronger, week after week, month after month, and year after year.

Swamped With Financial Opportunity Which He Turned Down

When he graduated from college he was swamped with financial opportunities, all of which he turned down in favor of becoming a community organizer in the midst of poverty, gangs, and drugs on the south side of Chicago where he personified optimism, intelligence, and relentless persistence to people who had been systematically beaten up, kicked around, chewed up, spit out, and generally rejected by the nation in which they lived.

In the Face of Scarcity, Gangs, Drugs, and Violence

And in the face of bitterness, cynicism, and anger he preached individual responsibility, strengthening oneself week after week, month after month, year after year. In the teeth of bigotry, injustice, racism and hatred, he preached relentless persistence. And in the bowels of scarcity, hunger, homelessness, gangs, drugs, and violence he preached "Oh Yes I Can" over and over and over again until people started to take him seriously. His relentless persistence became contagious, and small seeds of optimism were suddenly taking root in the belly of homes, neighborhoods, and precincts around the south side of Chicago.

Helping Others Grow Stronger Makes Him Stronger Yet

During this Chicago experience he discovered something very interesting. He found that when he helped others become stronger through relentless persistence his own strength grew and multiplied exponentially in a way that he'd never experienced before. In fact through these efforts he became so strong that he decided to run for public office in order to represent the relentlessly persistent group of people that was growing exponentially on the south side of Chicago.

44th President of the United States of America

First he ran for the local state legislature and became a member of the Illinois Senate. Then he ran for the United States Senate and he succeeded once again. And all the while he was doing battle with his mixed race background, his strange, un-American sounding name, and his big ears. But with relentless persistence and "Oh Yes I Can" he continued to become stronger by the week, the month, and the year..

So finally at age 47, with the world in a complete state of utter turmoil, he decided to run for the Presidency of the United States of America…while most Americans laughed, and many mocked or ignored him. But what they didn't know was that this new guy was absolutely overflowing with relentless persistence, and his "Yes We Can" message was contagious and it was precisely what America and the rest of the world needed to hear over and over and over again.

Simplistic, Idealistic, Yet Highly Instructional

Now you ask, is this a simplistic, even an idealistic portrait of the 44th President of the United States? I confess, yes it is. Has he fallen off the wagon on occasion? You betcha he has. Not only that, he's admitted as much in public, in black and white, in person, and in his books.

Defending a Government Of, By, and For the People

But the main thing is that he never fell far enough off the wagon that he failed to continue growing stronger and stronger, week after week, month after month, year after year. That's precisely why he is who he is, and why he's doing what he's doing.

And to the degree that our younger generation understands this simple formula and follows his lead, we'll be raising a generation of people who will themselves grow stronger week after week, month after month, year after year. And as the result that next generation will be strong, independent, self-reliant, and resilient enough to uphold and defend a legitimate democratic government of the people, by the people, and for the people. Yes, you could say it's all about RELENTLESS PERSISTENCE!! Yes we can.

An Open Letter to President Obama: How to Eliminate Childhood Obesity in One Decade or Less

Dear President Obama:

It's easy to help kindergartners learn how to do pull ups, and in the process to help them naturally immunize themselves against obesity for life by maintaining the ability to do pull ups. Yes, as most of us already know, kids who can do pull ups are never obese.

They're Natural Born Sponges

Why is it so easy you ask? Well, for starters, most kindergartners are natural born sponges when they first walk into school. They're already actively engaged in the process of soaking up the new experiences constantly swirling all around them, because it's natural, because it's novel and interesting, because they want to, and because real learning is FUN!

It's Fun

You see, at this age kids have yet to learn that education (in the adult sense) is actually an obligation not an opportunity. It's a job not a recreation. It's something they have to do not something they get to do. However, by second or third grade most of them have that one down in spades.

But, while they're still at this wide-eyed, bushy-tailed, soaking it up stage, it's easy to help kindergartners learn how to do pull ups, and they love every second of it because they all know you have to be strong in order to do pull ups. And there's not a kid on Planet Earth who doesn't want to be strong at everything and weak at nothing. It's in the genes.

Super-Sizing Has Yet to Take Root

The second reason it's easy to help kindergartners learn to do pull ups is that they have yet to have an opportunity to fully super-size themselves with bad eating and exercise habits. The older they get the greater the super-sizing odds become, and that puts kids in a rehabilitative rather than a preventative mode. Like anything else,

125

when it comes to childhood obesity, an ounce of prevention is worth a pound (billions of pounds) of cure every single day of the week.

Minimal Differences in Physical Efficiency

The third reason is that the difference in physical efficiency (body composition/ percentage of body fat) between boys and girls at this age is minimal. In fact in many cases the maturity of girls make them superior to boys when it comes to athletic activities like pull ups. It's always a mistake to sell the girls short in this strategy.

Huck, Tom, and Becky

With these thoughts in mind, consider the following scenario. Suppose we helped kindergarteners across the USA learn to do pull ups, and in the process to naturally immunize themselves against obesity for life, Tom, Huck, and Becky style.

Given access to a height adjustable pull up bar, and a technique called leg assisted pull ups, most kindergartners can easily develop this ability in one school year or less. That being the case, under the previous scenario, we'd have kindergartners across the USA who would avoid all the trials, tribulations, and expenses associated with childhood obesity, because they would have naturally immunized themselves against obesity at an early and impressionable age.

In Year Two

Now in year two we'd encourage and help the first group to maintain their newly developed ability, while introducing kindergarten class number two to same strength developing, confidence building, and obesity immunizing experiences that we introduced kindergarten class number one to the year before.

Childhood Obesity in the Rear View Mirror

If we continued with this strategy right on through high school, in a dozen years we'd be graduating class-full after class-full or high school seniors who could all physically pull their own weight and who are all naturally immunized against an insidious epidemic that a group of US Surgeon Generals has recently characterized as worse than smoking or Aids.

126

In reality my bet is that it would take less than a decade to fulfill this goal because it wouldn't take long before the kindergartners' older siblings caught wind of this new strength producing idea and would actively seek to become part of the growing movement. It would be considered COOL because, as we said before, all kids want to be strong at everything and weak at nothing... no matter how bad they claim to want to be.

In less than one decade, childhood obesity would be in the rear view mirror, something to read about in the history books like polio or the black plague. We'd have eliminated it once and for all.

Oh Yes We Can

Now as this nation enters this new age of YES WE CAN, what's stopping us from taking action and eliminating childhood obesity and related problems once and for all? Indications are that we're at a pivotal moment in our history. We're ready to turn the page, and to right old wrongs, moving on to a brighter future, so let's seize the day, carpe diem, and start eliminating childhood obesity in schools across the USA, and across the world.

We'll all sleep better at night knowing that we've finally done something that will make the world a better place for our kids and our grandkids. The best time to act is as always, RIGHT NOW!!!

Obama Takes the First Ever American Presidential Pull Your Own Weight Challenge...and Wins!

According to Time Magazine, when aides challenged him to a pull-up contest and each proceeded to do two pull-ups, Barack Obama proceeded to do three, and in the process he won the first ever American Presidential Pull Your Own Weight Challenge.

Interestingly enough taking the American Pull Your Own Weight Challenge seriously is one very simple and natural way to eliminate obesity from your life once and for all. In the words of one old coach "It doesn't matter if they're girls or guys, tall or short, rich or poor, black or white, Christian or Muslim. Show me ten people who can do pull-ups and I'll show you ten people who are NOT OBESE."

Immunizing Yourself Against Obesity for Life

You see, people who can do pull-ups are NEVER OBESE. And by combining a height adjustable pull-up bar with a technique called leg assisted pull-ups (jumping and pulling at the same time), almost anyone can learn to do pull-ups in a predictable amount of time. And once you've mastered the ability to do at least one pull-up (and more is always better), you've naturally IMMUNIZED YOURSELF against obesity FOR LIFE as long as you maintain the ability.

It Pays You for Two Things

More specifically, the pull-up bar pays you for two things. It pays you to be strong and it pays you to be light. The stronger you are and the lighter you are the more pull-ups you'll be able to do. On the other hand, the more pull-ups you can do, the stronger and lighter you have to be.

Thus in the process of learning and maintaining the ability to do pull-ups, the bar always pays you to eat right and exercise enough to do pull-ups. The ability to do pull-ups then serves as functional proof that you're eating well enough and getting enough exercise to naturally immunize yourself against obesity for life.

Stronger Week After Week, Month After Month

If you take a tip from Barack Obama and you get just a little bit stronger this week than you were last week, and a little bit stronger this month than last, you'll cultivate the habit known as Relentless Persistence, you'll be a lot stronger this year than you were last, you'll learn to pull your own weight, in the process you'll immunize yourself against obesity for life, and avoid all the problems associated with it.

Saluting the Purple Flag of Pull Your Own Weight

Whether you're a Democrat, a Republican, in a red state or a blue state (or an independent) we can all salute the purple flag of Pull Your Own Weight and eliminate obesity in America once and for all. And who knows, maybe one of these days you'll have a chance to win the Presidential Pull Your Own Weight Challenge just like Barack Obama. Yes you can!

Of Pull-ups, Childhood Obesity Prevention, and the Future of Democracy

Recently I saw a documentary movie in which an extraordinary old British gent contended that democracy is still the most revolutionary concept that the human race has ever encountered. He proceeded to observe that despotic governments manipulate and control their people by keeping them fearful, demoralized, and in debt.

Than he added, "Demoralized people don't vote, they don't take responsibility for themselves, and they don't maintain their right to a political democracy," he said. "You see it takes strong, healthy, resilient, self reliant, and self confident people to form and to maintain a democracy. Strong people are much harder to control than demoralized people." I found myself wanting to stand up in the audience in order to shout YES!!!!

OPYOW and Rugged Individualism

In that light I'd like to make the following comments about Operation Pull Your Own Weight, a program primarily focused on childhood obesity prevention, and on developing strong, resilient, self reliant kids who refuse to drink from the mass produced, conventional fountains of indoctrination. Above all else, these kids think for themselves.

There are those who have embraced OPYOW because of its ruggedly individualistic connotations, and I don't deny that rugged individualism is part of its appeal. We actively applaud strength, resilience, self-reliance, and personal responsibility taking behaviors. They are key components of being human in the fullest sense.

Social Darwinism VS Enlightened Self Interest

On the other hand, OPYOW is actively opposed to Social Darwinism, a theory that endorses a self centered, me first, to hell with you, survival of the fittest orientation to human existence. That may be part of American folklore, but in real life, self centered individualism all by itself is psychologically alienating and socially counterproductive.

Instead OPYOW favors enlightened self interest, a concept that takes the position "what's good for my family is good for me. And what's good for my neighborhood is good for my family. And what's good for my city, county, state, nation, world, is good for my neighborhood, my family, and me." In the words of some wise old man somewhere, "We're all in this together." Failing to understand and to act according to the principal of enlightened self interest undermines democracy.

OPYOW Salutes...

So does OPYOW salute rugged individuals who can fend for themselves, their family, their friends, and maybe even their city, state, nation, world? Absolutely! Does OPYOW salute rugged individuals who refuse the lure of conventional kool-aid and think for themselves? Without a doubt! And does OPYOW salute rugged individuals who use their strength to help strengthen others and help them to become confident, self reliant, yet also humble, mutually respectful, and therefore fully human? Yesiree Bob.

Egalitarianism, mutual respect, quiet self confidence, and enlightened self interest are at the heart of democracy and Operation Pull Your Own Weight. Hats off to both.

One is Never a Statistic

According to government sources the American taxpayer is spending over $120 billion dollars a year (the same as on the war in Iraq) on obesity and related problems and we're losing the war on all fronts. And all this is happening right here on American soil, not in Iraq, so there is no pulling out. We must stand and face the music!

The statistics, the odds, the medians, the percentages, and the averages related to this problem are growing more discouraging by the day. The problem is so rampant that the U.S. Surgeon General recently made Childhood Obesity Prevention his top priority, calling it "Terrorism from within." A forum of former US Surgeon Generals recently concluded that childhood obesity is a greater health threat than smoking or HIV Aids. The problem's getting worse not better.

Bad New VS Good News

But that's the bad news. Here's the good news. If you're reading this sentence you're not a pile of statistics, a median, a set of odds or averages, and neither are your kids. In fact personally I've never met or shaken hands with a statistic, an odd, or an average, which causes me question their validity, their legitimacy, their existence, and certainly their power over individual humans like you and me.

Strong, Resilient, Self Reliant

This essay then is intended to address real live parents, and real live educators, who have, work with, and care about real live kids, with real live challenges, and real live potential in dire need of cultivating, lest they live lives less than fully human. And if you reach them at a young enough age, there are very few of these real live kids who lack the innate talent to become strong, resilient, and self reliant human beings. In fact, truth be told, there are very few who lack the tools to become geniuses of one variety or another, if those talents are properly cultivated, and developed to their full potential.

Chuck The Experts

That being the case I say TO HECK WITH THE EXPERTS, their studies, their insidious webs of statistics, odds, and averages. Since their very existence is itself questionable, I suggest that they don't apply to you or your kids, or their friends.

They cannot prevent even one individual parent or educator from showing even one individual child how to get stronger, more resilient, and more self reliant (the only legitimate goal of education) on a weekly, monthly, and yearly basis. Nor can they prevent even one individual child from saying YES to, or from actively embracing those experiences that make them strong, resilient, and self reliant, happy, and fulfilled individuals.

From a philosophical standpoint, or even a religious perspective, there's a reason why kids are born to parents instead of to school systems. Parents and kids can become a family unit and can treat one another as unique, one-of-a-kind individuals, instead of mass produced products, a pile of statistics, a set of odds or averages. So I say cough up the conventional kool-aid, eliminate the indoctrinations, forget the experts, and when it comes to obesity prevention, take responsibility for yourself and your kids. Teach them how to physically Pull Their Own Weight. After all, ONE IS NEVER A STATISTIC.

Boiling it All Down Into One Simple Common Denominator

At the Risk of Pointing Out the Obvious...

1. Show me 10 boys who can do pull-ups and I'll show you 10 boys who are not obese. *

2. Show me 10 girls who can do pull-ups and I'll show you 10 girls who are not obese.

3. Show me 10 families full of members who can do pull-ups and I'll show you ten families who don't worry about obesity and all the related problems.

4. Show me an elementary or a high school full of students who can do pull-ups and I'll show you an elementary and a high school who've won the war on obesity.

5. Show me a school teacher, administrator, or a school board member who can do pull-ups and I'll show you a school teacher, an administrator, and a school board member who are all setting great examples for the kids in their schools to follow.

6. Show me a company (say McDonald's) full of employees who can do pull-ups and I'll show you a company that's healthy, energetic, productive, and inexpensive to insure.

7. Show me a police department whose members can do pull-ups and I'll show you a police department who doesn't worry about the relationship between cops and donuts.

8. Show me a group of childhood obesity prevention experts who can do pull-ups and I'll show you a group of childhood obesity prevention experts who walk the walk.

9. Show me a town/city, a county, a state, or a nation whose citizens can do pull-ups and I'll show you a town/city, a county, a state, and a nation who's won the war against obesity.

10. Show me a group of people who understand what you've just read here and I'll show you a group of people who are unconfused and ready to rally around "A simple, easily implemented, easily documented, and affordable solution to childhood obesity."

And Then, With a Straight Face...

1. Tell me why obesity prevention is so complicated and confusing that we're unable stop it from growing like a California forest fire raging out of control?

2. Tell me why every gym teacher in America agrees with the claim that kids who can do pull-ups are never obese, yet so few take the time to teach their kids to do pull-ups and to become obesity beating heroes in their own local communities at the same time?

3. Tell me why America's Surgeon General has named childhood obesity prevention his TOP PRIORITY yet to date has provided no actionable answers to the problem?

4. Tell me why the future and life quality of millions of boys and girls will be undermined and sacrificed by low self esteems due to ongoing battles with obesity?

5. Tell me why one large charitable organization (whose name I won't mention) has dedicated $500 million dollars over the next five years to defeating childhood obesity, yet after year one (one hundred million spent) they have so little to show for it?

6. Tell me why we're spending countless billions as a nation on obesity related illnesses?

7. Tell me why people in high positions simply fail to act, even when the obvious is pointed out to them?

8. Tell me why common sense is so uncommon, and why the obvious is so hard to see?

9. Tell me why we continue to think that the emperors are wearing beautiful and stylish new clothes when they're obviously standing stark naked in front of everyone, for anyone - with open eyes - to see?

10. And if this is true of an issue like childhood obesity prevention, doesn't it make you wonder how many other blatantly obvious solutions to crucial problems are being completely and totally overlooked and ignored by our so called authorities, our so called experts, our so called leaders?

(1) Substitute any sufficiently challenging functional acid test (i.e. dips, rope climbing, rock climbing, hand stand push ups, superman push ups) in place of pull-ups and the results will be the same.

A Form Letter for
Action Oriented People!

You could be a parent of a child who attends a particular school. You could be a teacher at that school. Or you could just be a local citizen or businessperson who's just plain fed up with <u>the total void</u> when it comes to taking any action against the problem of childhood obesity. So if you're sick and tired of all the talk, all the studies, all the research, and the billions that are being wasted on INACTION/TALK, this form letter is for you. Fill in the blanks with your own information, and send this letter out to the school principal, the superintendent of schools, and the local school board members in your home town and see if you can't stir up a little ACTION. Now check out the letter.

The Letter...

Dear _____:
    I know that childhood obesity is a very serious problem in the United States, and that many kids in our local school system show that we're no exception to the rule. So, as a member of this community and a concerned citizen, I'd like to start the ball rolling at _____ elementary school, and implement a strategy the American Society of Exercise Physiologists recently described as "A simple, easily implemented, easily documented, and affordable solution to childhood obesity."

Naturally Immunized Against Obesity for Life
    The idea is based on the common observation that kids/people who can do pull-ups are NEVER OBESE. It goes on to say that, if we start young, and give them access to the right information and the right equipment, there are very few kids who are unable to master pull-ups in a predictable amount of time. Furthermore, once they've learned to do pull-ups, these kids have <u>naturally immunized themselves against obesity for life</u>, as long as they maintain the ability to perform pull-ups.
    In simplest terms, kids who can do pull-ups can't be eating too poorly or else they'd be unable to do pull-ups. And kids who can

do pull-ups can't be under-exercising too much or else they too would be unable to do pull-ups. The ability to perform pull-ups thus serves as documented, functional proof that kids who can do them are eating well enough, and are getting enough exercise to avoid being obese. It's automatically built in.

My Five Year Plan

In any case, here's my five year plan. First, I volunteer to provide the necessary equipment, because it's affordable, and it takes up very little space. I'd like to start with all the kindergartners at _____ elementary school, and within one school year, I can guarantee that 90% will not only learn to do pull-ups, but they'll learn to look forward to the opportunity to get on the bar and to work at becoming a little stronger week after week, month after month, all year long. By the end of the school year 90% of the kindergartners in your school will have naturally immunized themselves against obesity for life, and the remaining 10% will be well on their way.

In year two we'll repeat the same scenario with the incoming kindergarteners, while making sure that last year's class (who are now first graders) maintain their hard won ability. We'll repeat this scenario over and over for five straight years, and by the time we're done you'll have an elementary school full of kids who can physically pull their own weight and who are all naturally immunized against obesity for life. If you continue to duplicate this scenario for 12 consecutive years you'll eliminate childhood obesity in this school district completely and totally in a dozen years.

Documented to the Hilt

One other point I'd like to make here. This project will be documented to the hilt right from the get go. That is to say for every child in the program we'll keep a performance chart that that will show the weekly progress (it's amazing how small increments of weekly progress motivate kids to want to do more) that he or she is making toward the desired goal of learning to do pull-ups by the end of the school year.

So if a parent wants to come in and see how their little Jimmy or Niclole is doing, we'll have everything we need in black and white, along with many reasons why they should encourage their kids to keep on keeping on. If a journalist drops in and wants to know what kinds of results this program is producing so they can tell the community all about it (which they most certainly will do), we'll have all the info right at our fingertips. Or if a school board member comes in and wants to see exactly what's going on so he/she can report back to their colleagues, just take out the charts, run off a few copies and they'll have everything they need to see to continue supporting the program.

A Pilot Program for Others to Learn From

This first year can serve as a pilot program from which the rest of the schools in our district can observe and learn. Once we've shown the way, other schools may want to join in and naturally immunize their own kids against obesity for life by helping them learn to physically pull their own weight in a predictable amount of time.

For that matter if you have other schools who'd like to be part of this initial pilot program, let me talk with them and explain how simple it is to immunize kids against obesity for life. If they're really action oriented people, they won't need any more in order to get started on their own program right away.

Done correctly we can become the model for schools across the USA, and show kids how easy it can be to immunize themselves against obesity for life. If this sounds interesting, please let me know when we can get together and discuss the details.

Thanks for your time and consideration, and I'll look forward to hearing back from you at your earliest convenience.

Sincerely,

Your Name
Your Address
Your Phone Number
Etc.

The Logistics of Operation Pull Your Own Weight

In school there are three potential settings for an Operation Pull Your Own Weight program including in the PE class, in the regular classroom, or in an after school, extracurricular setting. Let's check them out.

By its very nature OPYOW falls most naturally into the realm of the physical educator. By the same token (for a variety of reasons) since the most preventative time to start the program is in kindergarten, the simplest place to fit OPYOW into a curriculum is in the kindergarten classroom. And if it's impossible to fit into the PE class or the regular kindergarten class, OPYOW can also be plugged into the after school, club setting and still produce lots of kids who are naturally immunized against obesity for life.

Setting the Stage Effectively

Regardless of which setting you choose, I suggest that you kick things off by reading "*A Really Strong Story for Kids*" (found in a variety of places including on the Internet) to your kids in order to give them a context, and set the stage in a way that they'll understand what to expect before anyone does their first leg assisted pull-up.

At the end of the story make sure and ask the kids "Who wants to be strong at everything," and watch all the hands fly up. Then ask them "Who wants to be weak at anything," and watch NO hands fly up. With the story read and these two questions asked, you're ready to explain the mechanics of OPYOW and leg assisted pull-ups to your kids.

In the Physical Education Class

In the PE class, having 2, 3, or even 4 leg assisted pull-up stations will help you move things along and avoid bottlenecks. Working in rotating squads or even pairs will speed up the height adjustments and the record keeping. And whatever you do start each participant at a level where they can <u>EASILY PERFORM 8 REPS</u>.

How easy you ask? It should be so easy that each student will know beyond a shadow of a doubt that he/she can easily do 9 reps (just one more) in workout # 2.

Now in workout # 2 you ALLOW them to do 9 reps and NO MORE! In workout # 3 you allow them to do 10 reps and NO MORE. In workout # 4 you allow them to do 11 reps, in workout # 5 you allow them to do 12 reps, and in workout # 6 you RAISE THE BAR ONE INCH and repeat the entire 8 to 12 rep routine all over again for five more consecutive weeks (presuming two workouts per week and one set per workout).

Built in Pattern of Success

This strategy is specifically designed to insure that EACH CHILD WILL MAKE A LITTLE PROGRESS, get a little bit stronger, each and every time they touch the bar for at least 3 straight weeks, or six straight workouts. And if you set things up correctly you'll insure that your kids will use very small increments of change to make a little progress, in front of their friends, every single time they touch the bar for eight, ten, and even twelve straight weeks.

This initial stage of the program is intentionally designed to help your kids learn to EXPECT SUCCESS IN PUBLIC. And once they've learned to expect success, their odds of relentlessly persisting when the going gets tougher increases exponentially. And once you've built in a strong sense of relentless persistence their odds of learning to physically pull their own weight and naturally immunizing themselves against obesity for life also increases exponentially. Not only that, but the experience of wrestling first hand with a difficult task like pull-ups, persisting, and winning, will heavily influence the way your students tackle life in general.

Expect 90% of Your Kids to Be Immunized for Life

If you start the program at the beginning if the year with your kindergarten classes in the Physical Education class, you can expect at least 90% of your students to master the ability to perform pull-ups by the end of the school year, and the other 10% to be well on their way. In year two you repeat the same scenario with the new kindergarten students and make sure that last year's group (now first

141

graders) maintains their hard won ability, by allowing them to perform pull-ups at least once a week.

Eliminate Childhood Obesity in Your School System

If you repeat this scenario over and over again for five straight years you will have eliminated childhood obesity in your own elementary school. And if the strategy is carried on through junior high and high school, your school system will eliminate obesity in one decade or less, and you will be graduating kids who are dramatically more confident, more creative, more productive and whose life quality will be much better because of what you did with one group of kindergartners a decade ago.

In the Kindergarten Classroom

The kindergarten classroom is actually the simplest place to initiate an OPYOW program, and kindergarten teachers are always looking for ways to allow their kids to blow off a little excess energy. Presuming the teacher is game, you'll need to install a doorway pull-up bar to with you can attach a height adjustable bar or straps and create one simple workout station.

I suggest that instead of expecting yourself or the teacher to do the honors, you should consider asking the teacher to recruit a couple of parents to come in twice a week and put the kids through their paces. From my experience, once they get the hang of it, parents learn to look forward to this as much as the kids do. In this scenario you are still the overseer of the program, the person who needs to answer any questions. But with someone else doing the hands on part, you can cover multiple bases including your own class load and the OPYOW program simultaneously. Getting others involved and spreading the credit is always a good idea too.

OPYOW in the After School Club Setting

If conducting the program seems to be impossible in either the PE class or the kindergarten classroom, and you want to initiate an after school OPYOW club, then plan on spending 30 to 45 minutes after school, twice a week with the kids who want to learn to physically pull their own weight. The setting can now be in the gym, in any regular classroom, or even on the playground. Actually the OPYOW bar or the straps easily adapts to any swing set, so the playground is something to seriously consider if you're doing an after school edition.

Those Who are Willing to Take Action

One way or the other, if you'd like to make a real difference in the lives of kids, immunizing them against obesity for life is a great place to start. It's not expensive. It's not time consuming. But it does require educators who are willing to stand up and take action against a problem that's consuming a generation of kids. The real question is, are you one of those action oriented people? If so, the time to act is NOW.

More Thoughts on How to Organize A Pull Your Own Weight Program In Physical Education Class

If you are a physical education teacher, and want to do something significant and measurable to combat the growing problem of childhood obesity in this country, here's how you can help turn the tide, by following this suggested roadmap.

1. Start the year off by testing your students in a number of different functional fitness activities, but paying special attention to pull-ups.

2. Divide the students into two groups, those who can do at least one pull-up (group X), and those who can't do any pull-ups (group Y).

3. Then divide the students up into teams of equal size, and each team would be required to have at least one student who can do a pull-ups (from group X).

4. Make the student(s) from group X responsible for helping students from group Y learn to do pull-ups, and reward all successes with high fives, etc.

5. Create at least one (and probably three or four) height adjustable pull-up station, and show all students how to use the strategy of leg assisted pull-ups, "inching" their way up the chain until they eventually run out of leg assistance and can do regular pull-ups.

6. Introduce a story (Strong Food VS Weak Food) within which kids would understand good nutritional habits and monitor it according to progress on the pull-up bar.

7. Make sure that everyone from group X knows how to work correctly with their teammates from group Y.

8. Intentionally stack the deck by building small but regular successes (i.e. increasing reps by 1 each session) into the program for all participants.

9. Check out the possibility of having some intra-class, intra-grade, even intra-school competitions, being careful to <u>compare group to group</u> instead of individual student to individual student.

10. As far as individual students are concerned, encourage self-competition over competition with other students.

11. The first goal is to make sure that all participants make regular, tangible progress over a significant period of time...at least 12 weeks. This will establish a pattern of public success, and internalize motivation.

12. The primary, long term goal of course is to significantly increase the percentage of students who are members of group X from quarter to quarter, semester to semester, year to year, effectively immunizing kids against obesity for life.

13. Generate regular press releases (on school letterhead) so the local media is updated and would report regularly on how "we're attacking childhood obesity in our school."

14. Build a PYOW web-site so that the computer generation can check out all kinds of related things whenever they're on line.

15. Involve the private sector, many of whom are anxious to be identified with, even sponsor public educational success in a variety of ways.

16. Organize an annual Pull-Up-A-Thon between schools to help raise funds to benefit a worthwhile, local charity…such as childhood obesity prevention.

17. Try to track all kinds of related behaviors, including academic success.

18. Make it a privilege to participate. Forcing participation turns pull-ups into a job and effectively reduces its value to students.

19. Take advantage of the fact that all students want to be strong, not weak, and I'd cultivate a mentality favoring strength and independence over weakness and dependence.

20. Tell other physical educators about this program and encourage them to develop programs of their own for their own students.

21. Find companies in the area who'd like to sponsor PYOW employee wellness programs, and have students explain and design their program and get paid for doing it.

22. Find police and fire departments who'd like to participate and have students explain and design their program and get paid for doing it.

23. Find educators in schools who'd like to participate and have students explain and design their program and get paid for doing it.

24. Find parents who'd like to participate and have students design their program and pay them for it.

25. Go to city hall and recruit <u>politicians</u> who'd like to participate, etc.

26. Go to <u>park districts, Boy's and Girl's Clubs, YM/WCA's, Health Clubs, Pre-Schools, and churches,</u> to find out who else in the community would like to be able to physically Pull Their Own Weight, then encourage students to help them do so.

27. Encourage students to take pride in their peer's success, and I'll add more things to do when and if they come to me.

How Important is Confidence?

How important is confidence? In simplest terms, if you're in a situation where you're convinced that you can't succeed, you have no reason to even try. And when you don't try, the odds of succeeding are absolutely zero.

For example, <u>a citizen</u> who's convinced his vote doesn't count, has no reason to pay attention to politicians and to be informed in order cast an intelligent vote. Instead he simply tunes the whole thing out and stays home on election-day, which plays directly into the hands of those who want to dictate to and control others.

Or if <u>an unemployed person</u> is convinced that the market has no job for a person with their qualifications, they won't even bother to apply because it's a waste of time and effort. And when they fail to apply the odds of that unemployed person becoming a gainfully employed are zilch, zip, nada.

Or if <u>an investor</u> is totally convinced that investing in the current market is a losing proposition, he pulls his money out, sits in the sidelines, and refuses to participate. In other words the investor stops trying because he has NO CONFIDENCE in the market and the government agencies who are failing to regulate anything, while economic thugs are looting and pillaging the US economy. Yes, economically speaking the meltdown we're witnessing is the result of a complete and total COLLAPSE IN CONFIDENCE.

In the end confidence plays a significant role in anyone's ability to tackle difficult tasks successfully. Without confidence you don't try. And the minute you stop trying, failure is certain. That makes confidence pretty important.

The other important thing is to start teaching confidence right from the get go, and the best place to start is with a child's own physical body. In other words, kids who can handle themselves physically have a huge head start over kids who can't. That's where Operation Pull Your Own Weight comes in.

Just remember, all kids want to be strong at everything and weak at nothing. Help them fulfill that natural desire and confidence will follow along naturally in the wake.

Strong at Everything, Weak at Nothing...

Operation Pull Your Own Weight

The Five Goals

1. To compete with yourself, not others

2. To be stronger this week than last week

3. To be stronger this month than last month

4. To be stronger this year than last year

5. To learn to do pull-ups

The Seven Strength Generating Habits

1. Workout regularly

2. Eat right

3. Get sufficient rest

4. Avoid tobacco

5. Avoid alcohol

6. Avoid drugs

7. Take responsibility for doing these things yourself because nobody else can do them for you

The One Final Challenge

Once the seven habits are incorporated into your own life, the final challenge is to teach two others to do the same. Kids are inevitably amazed at how much stronger <u>THEY feel</u> after tackling and completing OPYOW's one final challenge.

The World is Shaped by Real People Who Take Action on Good Ideas

So you know a good idea when you see one, right? And Operation Pull Your Own Weight and naturally immunizing kids against obesity for life certainly qualifies as one of those good ideas whose time has come. Besides that, you're sick and tired of reading about the billions being spent on research, and the experts portraying childhood obesity as complicated, confusing and expensive when everyone knows that solving the problem is as simple as motivating kids to eat better and exercise more.

You clearly understand that done right, OPYOW is…
- Easy to understand
- Easy to implement
- Easy to document
- Extremely affordable for any school, park district, YMCA or Boys and Girls Club
- Naturally motivates kids to immunize themselves against obesity for life
- Improves life quality for millions of kids worldwide
- Saves taxpayers many billions annually

OK, if all that's true my question is what are you ready to do about it now? Are you inspired to take action now? Here's a brief list of things YOU could do NOW.
- Begin by initiating an OPYOW program in your own life and walking the walk.
- Introduce the idea to your own kids and encourage them to learn to PYOW
- Read the OPYOW book in order to get a thorough understanding of its potential
- Peruse the website for the same reasons
- Talk to a member of the local school board and introduce the idea
- Talk to a local PTA member and introduce the idea
- Write an op-ed piece for the local newspaper

- Gather of some of your local business associates and sponsor an OPYOW program in the local elementary schools who are interested in naturally immunizing their kids against obesity for life.
- Continue brainstorming with others and easily add 100 more good ideas to this list

It's one thing to recognize a good idea when you see one. But it's an entirely different matter to recognize a good idea, and to become inspired enough to take action on it. The world is full of people who recognize good ideas while standing idly by WAITING FOR SOMEONE ELSE to take action, ownership, and responsibility for making it happen. On the other hand the world is defined by those who pick the ball up themselves and run it across the goal line, or block for the guy doing the running, etc.

People Who are Willing to Take Action NOW!

So the question is, since you see what OPYOW can do for millions of kids around the world, what role are you willing to play in helping to make it happen?

If this note inspires you to take action then I am twice as strong as before you read it. And if you share it with your action oriented friends and colleagues we can multiply ourselves exponentially. And if we multiply ourselves exponentially we become a movement that is destined to eliminate childhood obesity in a decade or less. But it all depends on PEOPLE WHO ARE WILLING TO TAKE ACTION!

The OPYOW Pledge

With the goal of becoming a little bit stronger this week than last week, a little bit stronger this month than last month, and a lot stronger this year than last year...

I pledge to
- Workout two days each week
- For a maximum of 5 minutes/workout (10 minutes/ week)
- For one full year, or 52 straight weeks whichever comes first

Functionally and Physiologically Younger

As the result of this commitment I will expect not only to become stronger but to become functionally and physiologically younger week after week, month after month, for one entire year.

I Will Renew My Commitment

And if at the end of one full year I am significantly stronger, functionally and physiologically younger, I will renew my commitment for another year, year after year as long as I continue seeing significant progress.

Exponentially Stronger

And if the strategy lives up to its claims, I will commit to helping others discover what I've discovered and to take the Operation Pull Your Own Weight Pledge. And when and if I do, I also understand that I should expect to grow exponentially stronger as the result. In this light my strength potential is unlimited.

_____

Name and Date

The OPYOW Disclaimer

We fully recognize that <u>all exercises in which the participant's own body weight is the primary resistance factor</u> (functional work) benefit from fat loss (an excess workload reduction). That is to say, exercise activities such as push ups, sit ups, squats, dips, pull-ups, hand stand push ups jumping jacks, squat thrusts, walking, running, dancing, stair climbing will all improve with fat loss.

Not All Body Weight Exercises Qualify

However not all body weight exercises can predictably distinguish people who are obese apart from people who are not obese. In order to do that the body weight exercise must be sufficiently challenging.

So for example, jumping jacks don't qualify as predictors of obesity because some or many obese people can do jumping jacks. Dips on the other hand do qualify because those who can do them, can't be obese. Sit-ups don't qualify, but hand stand push ups do. Stair climbing doesn't qualify, but pull-ups do. In general, the more challenging the exercise, the more qualified and valuable it becomes as a predictor of obesity.

Another Variable

On the other hand, just because a participant is unable to perform pull-ups, dips, or hand stand push ups doesn't mean that they're obese. It's entirely possible for a person to be skinny (emaciated), weak, and lack the strength to do these kinds of challenging exercises. But people who are able to perform them are relatively lean and strong.

Here's Why We Chose Pull-ups

The main point here is, *we're not claiming that pull-ups have any corner on this functional acid test (FAT) orientation to obesity prevention.* But they're certainly one good example of it. The reason we chose pull-ups over all the others are threefold. First, most people know what pull-ups are. Second, pull-ups are inevitably associated with strength. And third, they line up so perfectly with the phrase Pull Your Own Weight.

Other Virtues

Other distinct virtues of pull-ups include the fact that they're extremely affordable, they require very little space to perform, and done right they're infinitely measurable. But if someone wanted to substitute dips, hand stand push ups, or a seven minute mile in place of pull-ups, you'd get no argument out of us at all.

www.ingramcontent.com/pod-product-compliance
Lightning Source LLC
Chambersburg PA
CBHW031207270326
41931CB00006B/457